Family Medicine

PreTest™ Self-Assessment and Review

Notice

Medicine is an ever-changing science. As new research and clinical experience broaden our knowledge, changes in treatment and drug therapy are required. The authors and the publisher of this work have checked with sources believed to be reliable in their efforts to provide information that is complete and generally in accord with the standards accepted at the time of publication. However, in view of the possibility of human error or changes in medical sciences, neither the authors nor the publisher nor any other party who has been involved in the preparation or publication of this work warrants that the information contained herein is in every respect accurate or complete, and they disclaim all responsibility for any errors or omissions or for the results obtained from use of the information contained in this work. Readers are encouraged to confirm the information contained herein with other sources. For example, and in particular, readers are advised to check the product information sheet included in the package of each drug they plan to administer to be certain that the information contained in this work is accurate and that changes have not been made in the recommended dose or in the contraindications for administration. This recommendation is of particular importance in connection with new or infrequently used drugs.

Family Medicine

PreTest™ Self-Assessment and Review
First Edition

Doug Knutson, MD
The Ohio State University

New York   Chicago   San Francisco   Lisbon   London   Madrid   Mexico City
Milan   New Delhi   San Juan   Seoul   Singapore   Sydney   Toronto

The **McGraw·Hill** Companies

Family Medicine: PreTest™ Self-Assessment and Review, First Edition

PreTest™ is a trademark of The McGraw-Hill Companies, Inc.

2 3 4 5 6 7 8 9 0   DOC/DOC   0 9 8

ISBN: 978-0-07-148269-1
MHID: 0-07-148269-5

This book was set in Berkeley by International Typesetting and Composition.
The editors were Laura K. Wenham and Regina Y. Brown.
The production supervisor was Sherri Souffrance.
Project management was provided by International Typesetting and Composition.
The cover designer was Maria Scharf.
Cover Photo: Blend Images Collection/Veer.com.
RR Donnelley was printer and binder.

This book is printed on acid-free paper.

Library of Congress Cataloging-in-Publication Data

Knutson, Doug (Douglas J.), 1962-
    Family medicine : pretest self-assessment and review / Doug Knutson.
      p. ; cm.
    Includes index.
    ISBN-13: 978-0-07-148269-1 (pbk. : alk. paper)
    ISBN-10: 0-07-148269-5 (pbk. : alk. paper)
    1. Family medicine—Examinations, questions, etc.
    [DNLM: 1. Family Practice—Examination Questions. WB 18.2 K67f   2008]
    I. Title.
    RC58.K58   2008
    610.76—dc22
                              2007026692

Student Reviewers

Shirley Ni
Ross University School of Medicine
Class of 2008

Anand Shah
University of Pennsylvania School of Medicine
Class of 2008

Kathryn Sulkowski
University of Medicine and Dentistry of New Jersey
School of Osteopathic Medicine
Class of 2007

Contents

Acknowledgments

I offer my heartfelt thanks to Cari Brackett, PharmD, and Kate Balturshot, MD, for help with some of the questions in this text. Additionally, I'd like to thank The Ohio State University Department of Family Medicine for the opportunities afforded to me. Most importantly, I'd like to thank John and Lucy for their support and encouragement.

An Introduction

Introduction

Family Medicine: PreTest Self Assessment and Review, First Edition, is intended to provide medical students, as well as house officers and physicians, with a convenient tool for assessing and improving their knowledge of medicine. The 500 questions in this book are similar in format and complexity to those included in Step 2, of the United States Medical Licensing Examination (USMLE). They may also be a useful study tool for Step 3.

Each question in this book has a corresponding answer, a reference to a text that provides background to the answer, and a short discussion of various issues raised by the question and its answer. A listing of references for the entire book follows the last chapter.

To simulate the time constraints imposed by the qualifying examinations for which this book is intended as a practice guide, the student or physician should allot about one minute for each question. After answering all questions in a chapter, as much time as necessary should be spent in reviewing the explanations for each question at the end of the chapter. Attention should be given to all explanations, even if the examinee answered the question correctly. Those seeking more information on a subject should refer to the reference materials listed or to other standard texts in medicine.

Preventive Medicine

Questions

Immunizations

1. You are examining a normal term newborn whose mother is hepatitis B virus surface antigen positive. Which of the following protocols is recommended for the child?

a. Hepatitis B vaccination at 0–2 months, a second dose at 1–4 months, and a third dose at 6–18 months of age

b. Hepatitis B vaccination within 12 hours of birth, with the timing of the second and third doses based on the mother's Hepatitis B viral load at the time of delivery

c. Hepatitis B vaccination and hepatitis B immune globulin within 12 hours of birth, a second dose of hepatitis B vaccine at 1–2 months, and a third dose of vaccine at 6 months

d. Hepatitis B vaccination and hepatitis B immune globulin within 12 hours of birth, a second dose of the vaccine and immune globulin at 1–2 months, and a third dose of the vaccine and immune globulin at 6 months

e. Hepatitis B vaccination at birth, with serologic testing of the baby before additional vaccinations are given

2. You are counseling a mother about her child's immunization schedule. She asks specifically if her child would benefit from the *Haemophilus influenzae* type b (Hib) vaccine. Which of the following statements is true about this vaccine?

a. The vaccine is between 95–100% effective in preventing invasive Hib disease

b. The vaccine will help to prevent otitis media caused by *H. influenzae*

c. Adverse reactions to the vaccine include an unusual high-pitched cry, high fevers, and seizures

d. The first vaccine should be administered at birth

e. The vaccine cannot be given concurrently with other vaccines

3. You are discussing varicella-zoster vaccination with an adult who does not ever remember having chicken pox. Which of the following statements is true?

a. Varicella-zoster infection is less severe in adults
b. The varicella vaccine is less immunogenic in adults
c. Serologic testing for varicella antibodies is necessary before vaccination
d. If the patient lives with an immunocompromised person, vaccination should be avoided
e. The subsequent risk of zoster is higher among those who have been vaccinated as compared with those who had natural infection

4. An elderly patient that you follow has recently started hemodialysis for chronic renal failure. You know that hepatitis B vaccination is recommended for people on hemodialysis, and find that he is hepatitis B surface antibody negative. Which of the following would be the best guideline to follow in this case?

a. No vaccination is necessary based on his laboratory evaluation
b. Administer one dose of hepatitis B vaccine
c. Administer two doses of hepatitis B vaccine, at least 1 month apart
d. Administer two doses of hepatitis B vaccine, at least 6 months apart
e. Administer three does of hepatitis B vaccine at the appropriate time interval

5. You are caring for a 23-year-old healthy homosexual male who works as an accountant and lives alone. He had the "typical childhood vaccinations" and provides documentation of his immunization record. He is up to date on tetanus, and was primarily immunized against diphtheria, pertussis, polio, hepatitis B, measles, mumps, rubella, and *H. influenzae* type b. Which of the following vaccinations is indicated for this patient?

a. Varicella
b. Meningococcus
c. Hepatitis A
d. Pneumococcus
e. A booster of the measles, mumps, and rubella (MMR) vaccine

6. In the prenatal workup for one of your patients, you discover she is rubella nonimmune. When is the best time to vaccinate the patient against rubella?

a. Immediately
b. In the second trimester of pregnancy
c. In the third trimester of pregnancy
d. In the early postpartum period
e. At least 4 weeks postpartum

7. An adult is seen in your office after cutting her hand on a clean broken glass in her kitchen. She received her primary tetanus series as a child. The wound is relatively minor, and does not require suturing. Her last tetanus booster was 7 years ago. Which of the following is true?

a. No vaccination is required
b. The patient should receive a tetanus-diphtheria (Td) booster
c. The patient should receive a Td booster and tetanus immune globulin
d. The patient should receive a diphtheria-tetanus-pertussis (DTP) booster
e. The patient should receive a diphtheria-tetanus-acellular pertussis (DTaP) booster

8. You are caring for a woman who would like her children vaccinated against influenza. Her children are ages 4 months, 24 months, and 5 years. Which of the following represents current immunization recommendations for influenza?

a. None of her children should be vaccinated
b. The 4-month-old and the 24-month-old should be vaccinated
c. The 24-month-old and the 5-year-old should be vaccinated
d. Only the 24-month-old should be vaccinated
e. All the children should be vaccinated

Screening Tests

9. You are discussing preventive health screening with a college student. He has no family history of hypertension, coronary artery disease, diabetes, or cancer. At what age would you consider screening for lipid disorders?

a. 18 years
b. 21 years
c. 25 years
d. 35 years
e. 50 years

10. You are seeing a 58-year-old smoker for a routine health examination. You have counseled him on discontinuing tobacco use, and he is considering that alternative. He denies coughing, shortness of breath, or hemoptysis. Which of the following is a recommended screen for lung cancer in this patient?

a. He should not be screened for lung cancer
b. Chest x-ray
c. Chest CT
d. Sputum cytology
e. Bronchoscopy

11. You are seeing a healthy 26-year-old woman for a routine health visit. She mentions that she and her husband are thinking about starting a family soon. She has never been pregnant before. Which of the following interventions has been shown to have a clear beneficial outcome at this time?

a. Blood typing and antibody testing
b. Screening for human immunodeficiency virus (HIV)
c. Screening for Chlamydia
d. Screening for asymptomatic bacteriuria
e. Prescribing 0.4–0.8 mg of folic acid daily

12. You are discussing cancer screening with a patient. Her father was diagnosed with colorectal cancer at age 72. When should you recommend she begins colorectal cancer screening?

a. 40 years
b. 50 years
c. 60 years
d. 62 years
e. 72 years

13. You are discussing cancer screening with a female patient. She has no family history of breast cancer. At what age should she start getting routine mammograms?

a. 30
b. 35
c. 40
d. 45
e. 50

14. In a routine examination, a 33-year-old woman asks you about self-breast examination as breast cancer screening method. Which of the following best represents current recommendations for breast self-examination (BSE)?

a. There is strong evidence that BSE is an appropriate screening modality
b. There is no evidence that BSE is an appropriate screening modality
c. There is insufficient evidence to recommend for or against BSE
d. There is no evidence that BSE is an inappropriate screening modality
e. There is strong evidence that BSE is an inappropriate screening modality

15. A 52-year-old man comes to your office for a complete physical examination. He is interested in prostate cancer screening. Which of the following best represents current guidelines for prostate cancer screening?

a. No screening guidelines are recommended
b. Screening should consist of a digital rectal examination
c. Screening should consist of a serum prostate specific antigen (PSA) test
d. Screening should consist of both a digital rectal examination (DRE) and a serum PSA test
e. Screening should include a computed tomography (CT) scan of the prostate in high-risk individuals

16. You are seeing a 40-year-old healthy man for a routine health examination. He is completely healthy, takes no medications, and has no abnormal physical examination findings. What are the current recommendations regarding obtaining a screening electrocardiogram (ECG) as part of his routine physical?

a. Recommendations strongly support obtaining a screening ECG
b. Recommendations weakly support obtaining a screening ECG
c. Recommendations do not support or oppose obtaining a screening ECG
d. Recommendations weakly oppose obtaining a screening ECG
e. Recommendations strongly oppose obtaining a screening ECG

17. During an appointment to discuss acne, you find that your 16-year-old female patient has become sexually active. According to current guidelines, when should you begin cervical cancer screening on this patient?

a. At the current time
b. At the age of 18
c. At the age of 19
d. At the age of 21
e. Cervical cancer screening is not recommended

18. You are seeing a 55-year-old patient for her annual physical examination. She has been married to her husband for 32 years and has never had sex with anyone else during the marriage. She has never had an abnormal Papanicolaou (Pap) smear. At what age is it appropriate to discontinue Pap screening on this patient?

a. 55 years old
b. 60 years old
c. 65 years old
d. 70 years old
e. Never discontinue screening

The Preoperative Evaluation

19. A 76-year-old male patient of yours is undergoing a left knee replacement for severe arthritis, and you are asked to perform his presurgical clearance. His past medical history is significant for episodic rate-controlled atrial fibrillation, a stroke at age 72 (from which he recovered fully), and uncontrolled hypertension. Last year, an echocardiogram showed he had severe aortic stenosis, but he has elected not to undergo surgical repair. He reports that he is sedentary, and is not able to walk up one flight of steps carrying his groceries without stopping to rest. His blood pressure upon evaluation is 168/92. Which of the described features are clinical predictors of increased perioperative cardiovascular risk for this surgery?

a. Advanced age
b. Rate-controlled atrial fibrillation
c. Uncontrolled hypertension
d. Severe aortic stenosis
e. Poor functional capacity

20. You are concerned about the cardiac risks of several of your patients undergoing surgical procedures, and are considering further cardiac testing in the preoperative period. Which of the following surgical procedures is considered to have a low surgery-specific risk, and generally does not require additional preoperative cardiac testing, if the patient does not have clinical predictors of increased cardiac risk?

a. Femoral-popliteal bypass
b. Breast surgery
c. Thyroidectomy
d. Knee replacement
e. Carotid endarterectomy

21. You are doing a preoperative history and physical examination on a 58-year-old woman who will be undergoing a cholecystectomy later in the month. She is obese, sedentary with type 2 diabetes, hyperlipidemia and a history of congestive heart failure in the past. She reports that she is unable to walk four blocks without stopping to rest. She denies chest pain with activity. Which of her historical features is *not* a risk factor for adverse postoperative outcomes?

a. Obesity
b. Functional capacity

c. Type 2 diabetes
d. Hyperlipidemia
e. Congestive heart failure

22. You are doing a routine preoperative clearance for an otherwise healthy 60-year-old man undergoing a knee replacement. Which of the following laboratory tests should be ordered?

a. Hemoglobin
b. Electrolytes
c. Blood glucose
d. Serum creatinine
e. Urinalysis

23. A 50-year-old male patient is presenting for preoperative testing before undergoing arthroscopic knee surgery. Which of the following is true regarding ordering a preoperative ECG for this patient?

a. The patient should have a preoperative ECG done regardless of history or physical examination
b. The patient should have a preoperative ECG done if he has a family history of hypertension
c. The patient should have a preoperative ECG done if he has a family history of coronary artery disease
d. The patient should have a preoperative ECG done if he is found to have elevated blood pressure during the preoperative evaluation
e. The patient should have a preoperative ECG done if he has a history of tobacco use

Travel Medicine

24. You are counseling one of your patients who is planning a trip overseas. He is concerned about becoming ill while traveling. Which of the following illnesses is the most common seen in international travelers?

a. Diarrhea
b. Upper respiratory infection
c. Parasitic infection
d. Malaria
e. Hepatitis

25. You are counseling a patient who is planning a trip with his wife to celebrate their 30th anniversary. They are going on an African Safari, and wonder about health risks associated with international travel. What would you tell him is the most common cause of death among international travelers?

a. Infections
b. Accidents
c. Homocide
d. Heart disease
e. Vascular disease (i.e., deep venous thrombosis and pulmonary embolus)

26. You are performing a physical examination on a student traveling to Mexico with her college Spanish class. She is concerned about traveler's diarrhea, and asks about antibiotic prophylaxis. Which of the following best represents the current guideline from the Centers for Disease Control (CDC) for prevention of traveler's diarrhea?

a. The CDC does not have an antibiotic guideline regarding antibiotic prophylaxis for traveler's diarrhea
b. Trimethoprim-Sulfamethoxazole
c. Doxycycline
d. Ciprofloxacin
e. Metronidazole

27. You are discussing vaccinations for a patient who is traveling internationally. Due to a significant fear of needles, he is unwilling to obtain any vaccination unless he feels there is significant risk of acquiring the condition. Which of the following vaccine preventable illness is the most common one acquired by travelers?

a. Yellow fever
b. Polio
c. Hepatitis A
d. Cholera
e. Typhus

28. One of your patients is a medical student planning a mission trip to equatorial Africa. He is asking about the yellow fever vaccine and the risks of complications from the vaccine. Which of the following is true regarding yellow fever vaccination?

a. The yellow fever vaccine is a killed vaccine, and therefore has minimal associated side effects
b. The yellow fever vaccine is a live vaccine, and does not have clinically significant risks associated with its use
c. The complications associated with the vaccine are rarer than the risk of developing yellow fever in equatorial Africa
d. The risk of yellow fever vaccine associated encephalitis is higher than the risk of becoming infected with yellow fever, therefore vaccination is not recommended
e. The risk of developing a syndrome resembling wild-type yellow fever after vaccination is higher than the risk of becoming infected with yellow fever, therefore vaccination is not recommended

29. You are discussing required vaccinations for an HIV infected traveler. Which of the following vaccines is recommended for immunodeficient patients?

a. Yellow fever vaccine
b. Inactivated polio vaccine
c. Cholera vaccine
d. Oral typhoid vaccine
e. MMR vaccine

Contraception

30. You are re-evaluating a 32-year-old woman in your office. You started her on combination oral contraceptives (COCs) 3 months ago, and at each of three visits since then, her blood pressure has been elevated. Which of the following is an appropriate next step?

a. Discontinue the oral contraceptive and recommend a barrier method
b. Change to a pill with a higher estrogen component
c. Change to a pill with a lower estrogen component
d. Change to a pill with a lower progestin component
e. Change to a progestin-only pill

31. Which side effect of COCs is most frequently cited as the reason for discontinuing their use?

a. Nausea
b. Breast tenderness
c. Fluid retention
d. Headache
e. Irregular bleeding

32. You are counseling a 23-year-old woman who is interested in starting COC pills. Which of the following is true regarding risks associated with COC use?

a. Users of COC pills have an increased risk of ovarian cancer
b. Users of COC pills have an increased risk of endometrial cancer
c. Users of COC pills have an increased risk of thromboembolism
d. Users of COC pills have an increased risk of hemorrhagic stroke
e. Users of COC pills have an increased risk of diabetes mellitus

33. A 29-year-old obese woman with type 2 diabetes mellitus is asking you about progestin-only pills as a method of contraception. Which of the following is true?

a. Progestin-only pills are contraindicated in women with diabetes
b. Progestin-only pills would increase her risk of thromboembolic events
c. Progestin-only pills are only Food and Drug Administration (FDA) approved for nursing women
d. Progestin-only pills increase her risk for ectopic pregnancy
e. Progestin-only pills should be taken every day of the month, without a hormone-free period

34. You are counseling a patient regarding contraception options. She is 36-years-old, she smokes, weighs 145 lb, and has no other medical concerns. She is sexually active, but not in a monogamous relationship. Of the following, which is her best contraception option?

a. Combination oral contraceptive pills
b. An intravaginal ring system delivering estrogen and progestin
c. A transdermal contraceptive patch delivering estrogen and progestin
d. An injectable form of long-acting progestin
e. An intrauterine device (IUD)

35. A 28-year-old monogamous married woman comes to you for emergency contraception. She and her husband typically use condoms to prevent pregnancy, but when they had sex 2 evenings ago, the condom broke. She does not want to start a family at this time. Which of the following statements is true regarding the use of emergency contraception pills (ECPs)?

a. She is too late to use ECPs in this case
b. ECPs are 90–100% effective when used correctly
c. There are no medical contraindications to the use of ECPs, other than allergy or hypersensitivity to the pill components
d. ECPs disrupt the pregnancy, if given within days of implantation
e. Clinicians should perform a pregnancy test before prescribing ECPs

Preventive Medicine

Answers

1. The answer is c. (*South-Paul, pp 78–93.*) Hepatitis B infection is more likely to become chronic when acquired early in life. In 1991, the CDC recommended universal immunization of infants in the United States. The vaccine is given in a three-dose schedule, with the timing dependent on the mother's hepatitis B surface antigen status. If the mother is hepatitis B surface antigen positive, the first dose of vaccine and a dose of hepatitis B immune globulin must be given within 12 hours of birth. The second dose of vaccine is given at 1–2 months, and the third dose is given at 6 months. For mothers with unknown antigen status, the first dose of vaccine should be given within 12 hours, and maternal blood should be drawn to determine status. If the mother's surface antigen is positive, the child is given immune globulin as soon as possible, but no later than 1 week of age. For mothers with negative antigen status, the first dose of vaccine is given at 0–2 months, the second at 1–4 months, and the third at 6–18 months.

2. The answer is a. (*South-Paul, pp 78–93.*) Before the introduction of an effective vaccine, Hib caused invasive disease in about 1 of every 200 children in the United States. Hib meningitis was the most common invasive Hib illness, carried a 2–5% mortality rate, even with appropriate treatment, and up to 30% of survivors developed neurological sequelae. In the first 10 years of the vaccine's use, the incidence of invasive Hib disease decreased 97%. The vaccine does not reduce the rate of otitis media, as most cases are due to nontypeable *H. influenzae*. Adverse reactions to the vaccine are very rare. In fact, no serious reactions have been linked to the vaccine. The vaccine should not be administered before 6 weeks of age, as immune tolerance to the antigen may be induced. The vaccine may be given with other vaccines.

3. The answer is b. (*South-Paul, pp 78–93.*) Varicella-zoster infection is more severe in neonates and adults. The vaccine is less immunogenic in those over the age of 13, and therefore two doses of vaccine are required, given 4–8 weeks apart. While many people who do not remember having chicken pox have serologic evidence of immunity, testing is not necessary, as the vaccine is well-tolerated in those already immune. No special precautions are necessary for households with immunocompromised persons, unless the person vaccinated develops a rash. Zoster is more common among those with natural infection as opposed to those who were immunized.

4. The answer is e. (*Rakel, pp 182–193.*) Hepatitis B vaccination is recommended for nonimmune people who are high risk. Those include men who have sex with men, people with multiple sexual partners, sex industry workers, intravenous drug users, prison inmates, people on hemodialysis, people living in households with hepatitis B virus carriers, health care workers and people from endemic areas. In this question, having surface antibody negativity means that the patient has never been exposed and is nonimmune. The immunization schedule is one injection at time 0, one between 1–2 months after that, and a third injection between 4–6 months after the second.

5. The answer is c. (*Rakel, pp 182–193.*) Hepatitis A vaccination is indicated for men who have sex with men or users of illegal drugs. The patient is not at high risk for varicella, and therefore vaccination is not indicated. Meningitis vaccination is indicated for those with functional asplenia or travelers to endemic areas. College students can be counseled about the vaccination, especially if they are living in a dormitory. Pneumococcal vaccination is only indicated for those with chronic diseases, functional asplenia or residents of long term care facilities. An MMR booster is not indicated.

6. The answer is d. (*Rakel, pp 182–193.*) Congenital rubella syndrome is devastating, and rubella immunity is important for women considering pregnancy. If a woman is found to be rubella nonimmune, vaccination should not occur if she is pregnant or planning pregnancy in the next 4 weeks. If she is currently pregnant and nonimmune, she should be vaccinated as early in the postpartum period as possible.

7. The answer is a. (*Mengel, pp 712–724.*) Adults should receive a Td booster every 10 years. Booster shots are not required for clean, minor wounds. For contaminated or deep wounds, a booster is recommended if the last vaccination was given more than 5 years ago. If the immunization history is unclear, tetanus immune globulin may be indicated for a contaminated wound. DTP and DTaP are not recommended in adults.

8. The answer is c. (*Rakel, pp 182–193.*) Influenza vaccination is recommended annually for children ages 6 months and greater with certain risk factors (asthma, cardiac disease, sickle cell disease, HIV, and diabetes among others). It can be administered to all others wishing to obtain immunity as well. In addition, children between 6–24 months should be offered the vaccine, as they are at substantial risk for hospitalization if infected. In this case, since the mother wishes all her children be vaccinated, only the 4-month-old should be excluded because of age.

9. The answer is d. Determining which screening tests are appropriate for a patient is difficult, and requires individual judgment based on the clinical situation. The American Academy of Family Physicians has developed clinical preventive services charts based on age alone in low-risk adults, and rank the screen as "strongly recommend," "recommend," and "healthy behavior." Strongly recommended screens are supported by good quality evidence and demonstrate substantial net benefit for the patient. It is strongly recommended that men are screened for lipid disorders at age 35 even in the absence of other risk factors. Screening would occur earlier in the presence of diabetes, a family history of heart disease by age 50, or with other risk factors.

Recommendations for clinical preventative services. The American Academy of Family Physicians. Available at http://www.aafp.org/online/en/home/clinical/exam/ko.html. Accessed October 3, 2006.

10. The answer is a. The U.S. preventive services task force has found that CT scanning, chest x-ray, and sputum cytology can detect lung cancer at an earlier stage than no screening at all, but also found no evidence that any screening strategy actually improves mortality. Therefore, no screening is recommended for this patient.

Recommendations for clinical preventative services. The American Academy of Family Physicians. Available at http://www.aafp.org/online/en/home/clinical/exam/ko.html. Accessed October 3, 2006.

11. The answer is e. Of the interventions listed above, only prescribing folic acid has been shown to be beneficial prior to pregnancy. It will decrease the chance of neural tube defects in the baby. The other interventions should be done early in the pregnancy to ensure good pregnancy outcome.

Recommendations for clinical preventative services. The American Academy of Family Physicians. Available at http://www.aafp.org/online/en/home/clinical/exam/ko.html. Accessed October 3, 2006.

12. The answer is b. In general, colorectal cancer screening should begin at age 50. In cases where there is a family history of colorectal cancer, the screen should begin 10 years before the cancer was diagnosed in the family, or at age 50, whichever is sooner.

Recommendations for clinical preventative services. The American Academy of Family Physicians. Available at http://www.aafp.org/online/en/home/clinical/exam/ae.html. Accessed October 3, 2006.

13. The answer is c. Mammograms (with or without clinical breast examinations) have clearly been shown to reduce mortality associated with breast cancer. Guidelines vary, but the U.S. Preventative Services Task Force recommends routine mammography every 1–2 years beginning at age 40.

Recommendations for clinical preventative services. The American Academy of Family Physicians. Available at http://www.aafp.org/online/en/home/clinical/exam/ae.html. Accessed October 3, 2006.

14. The answer is c. The American Academy of Family Physicians has concluded that there is insufficient evidence to recommend for or against using BSE as a screening modality. Evidence is poor that BSE reduces mortality, and there is fairly strong evidence that BSE is associated with an increased risk for false-positive results and biopsies. Due to limitations in published and ongoing studies, the balance between benefits and harm is not known.

Recommendations for clinical preventative services. The American Academy of Family Physicians. Available at http://www.aafp.org/online/en/home/clinical/exam/ae.html. Accessed October 3, 2006.

15. The answer is a. There is evidence supporting DRE and PSA testing as a prostate cancer screen, but concerns exist regarding false positive tests and any actual reduction in mortality that is gained from doing the tests. Therefore, the American Academy of Family Physicians feels the evidence is insufficient to recommend for or against routine prostate cancer screening. In patients who are interested in screening, physicians should discuss the potential benefits and harms with the patients before making a decision to test.

Recommendations for clinical preventative services. The American Academy of Family Physicians. Available at http://www.aafp.org/online/en/home/clinical/exam/pt.html. Accessed October 3, 2006.

16. The answer is e. The American Academy of Family Physicians recommends against the routine use of the ECG as part of periodic health or preparticipation examinations in asymptomatic adults. There is no evidence that the use of ECG screening improves mortality or identification of asymptomatic disease.

Recommendations for clinical preventative services. The American Academy of Family Physicians. Available at http://www.aafp.org/online/en/home/clinical/exam/ae.html. Accessed October 3, 2006.

17. The answer is c. There is a strong recommendation from the American Academy of Family Physicians for cervical cancer screening at least every 3 years for women who have ever had sex and have a cervix. However, the optimal age at which to begin screening is unknown. Some recommend that screening should start at the onset of sexual activity or at age 18, whichever comes first. However, evidence, coupled with the natural history of HPV infection, indicates that screening can safely be delayed until 3 years after the onset of sexual activity or age 21, whichever comes first.

Recommendations for clinical preventative services. The American Academy of Family Physicians. Available at http://www.aafp.org/online/en/home/clinical/exam/ae.html. Accessed October 3, 2006.

18. The answer is a. Guidelines for low-risk women indicate that Pap testing should be conducted at least every 3 years in women who have ever had sex and still have a cervix. The guidelines regarding when to discontinue testing are not as clear. However, the yield of the Pap test is low in women who have been previously screened at age 65. The American Cancer Society recommends discontinuing screening at age 70, but also notes that a woman who has had three or more documented normal, technically satisfactory Pap tests, and has had no abnormal Pap tests in the last 10 years can safely stop screening.

Recommendations for clinical preventative services. The American Academy of Family Physicians. Available at http://www.aafp.org/online/en/home/clinical/exam/ae.html. Accessed October 3, 2006.

19. The answer is d. Family physicians are often asked to perform preoperative evaluations for their patients. The purpose of these evaluations is to identify risks for poor outcomes that may not be immediately apparent to the surgeon. In 2002, the American College of Cardiology and the American Heart Association summarized clinical predictors for increased perioperative cardiovascular risk. They found that advanced age, a rhythm other than sinus rhythm (atrial fibrillation), uncontrolled hypertension and low functional capacity were not proven to independently increase perioperative cardiovascular risk in low or intermediate risk surgeries. However, severe heart valve disease was a major predictor of perioperative risk. Other major predictors are acute myocardial infarction (MI) (within 7 days), recent MI (between 8–30 days), unstable or severe angina, decompensated heart failure, high grade A/V block, symptomatic arrhythmias with underlying heart disease, and supraventricular arrhythmias with a poorly controlled ventricular rate.

Shammash JB, Kimmel SE, Morgan JP. Estimation of cardiac risk prior to noncardiac surgery. Available at http://www.utdol.com/utd/content/topic.do?topicKey=periart/7170&type=A&selectedTitle=6~58. Accessed December 3, 2006.

20. The answer is b. When evaluating a patient's risk for undergoing a surgical procedure, the family physician must look at the patient-specific clinical variables, the patient's exercise capacity, and the risk of the surgical procedure being performed. High-risk surgical procedures are those with a risk of cardiac death greater than 5%, and include emergent operations, aortic or other major vascular surgeries, peripheral artery surgery, or prolonged surgeries with large anticipated fluid shifts. Intermediate risk procedures have a risk of cardiac death between 1–5% and include carotid endarterectomies, head and neck surgeries, intrathoracic and intraperitoneal surgeries, orthopedic surgeries and prostate surgeries. Low risk procedures have a risk of cardiac death less than 1% and generally do not require additional cardiac preoperative testing. They include endoscopic procedures, superficial procedures, cataract surgeries, and breast surgery.

Shammash JB, Kimmel SE, Morgan JP. Estimation of cardiac risk prior to noncardiac surgery. Available at http://www.utdol.com/utd/content/topic.do?topicKey=periart/7170&type=A&selectedTitle=6~58. Accessed December 3, 2006.

21. The answer is a. Surprisingly, obesity is not a risk factor for adverse postoperative outcomes. Type 2 diabetes, hyperlipidemia, and congestive heart failure may all require additional preoperative testing. Poor functional capacity is defined as being unable to walk four blocks or up two flights of steps. Persons with poor functional capacity have more than twice as many adverse outcomes than their counterparts with better functional capacity.

Smetana GW. Preoperative medical evaluation of the healthy patient. Available at http://www.utdol.com/utd/content/topic.do?topicKey=med_cons/6474&view=print. Accessed November 30, 2006.

22. The answer is d. Random preoperative laboratory testing can increase costs, have little benefit, and a high rate of false-positive tests. Therefore, selective use of laboratory tests is a more prudent approach. In general, guidelines suggest a hemoglobin or hemotacrit for surgery with expected major blood loss and electrolytes only if the patient has a history that increases the likelihood of an abnormality (diuretic use). Routine blood glucose and urinalysis measurements are not recommended. Serum creatinine should be tested if the surgery is major, hypotension is expected, nephrotoxic drugs will be used or the patient is above 50.

Smetana GW. Preoperative medical evaluation of the healthy patient. Available at http://www.utdol.com/utd/content/topic.do?topicKey=med_cons/6474&view=print. Accessed November 30, 2006.

23. The answer is a. Most experts agree that a preoperative ECG should be performed routinely in:

- Men older than 45 years
- Women older than 55 years
- Patients with a history of known cardiac disease
- Patients with a clinical history suggesting cardiac disease
- Patients at risk for electrolyte abnormalities, such as those using diuretics
- Patients with systemic disease associated with unrecognized cardiac disease, such as hypertension or diabetes
- Patients undergoing major surgical procedures

In the case above, the patient's age indicated he would have an ECG regardless of the other factors identified in the history or physical.

Smetana GW. Preoperative medical evaluation of the healthy patient. Available at http://www.utdol.com/utd/content/topic.do?topicKey=med_cons/6474&view=print. Accessed November 30, 2006.

24. The answer is a. (*Rakel, pp 193–204.*) Approximately 50 million people travel abroad each year. Of these, almost 50% will become ill while traveling. Traveler's diarrhea is the most common illness, followed by upper respiratory infection (URI), viral syndromes, skin conditions, parasitic infections, malaria, hepatitis, and other more rare infections.

25. The answer is d. (*Rakel, pp 193–204.*) Heart disease is the most common cause of death while traveling, likely because it is such a common cause of death in general. The second most common cause of death is accidents. People traveling engage in risky behavior that they otherwise might not while on vacation. Dangerous recreation activities, increased drinking, driving in foreign countries all contribute to causing accidents. Discussing accident prevention is therefore the key when counseling patients planning to travel abroad.

26. The answer is a. (*Rakel, pp 193–204.*) The CDC does not recommend antibiotic chemoprophylaxis for traveler's diarrhea because of the development of resistant organisms. Most times, the condition is self-limited. The CDC does recommend using common sense regarding food and water, eating nothing unless it is boiled, peeled, or cooked.

27. The answer is c. (*Rakel, pp 193–204.*) Hepatitis A is the most common vaccine preventable illness acquired by travelers. Yellow fever is the only legally required immunization (and then, only for some countries). A single inactivated polio vaccine (IPV) booster is recommended for adult travelers who have had primary polio immunization, but who will be traveling to an area where polio is endemic. Cholera and typhus are generally not required immunizations for travelers.

28. The answer is c. Yellow fever is a mosquito-borne viral infection and is endemic in equatorial Africa and areas of South America. Two rare complications of yellow fever can occur—encephalitis, and a syndrome resembling wild-type yellow fever. The risk of developing yellow fever for the unvaccinated traveler is 1 in 1000 while the risk of complication is 2.5–6 per 1 million vaccinations.

Weller PF. Immunizations for travel. Available at http://www.utdol.com/utd/content/topic.do?topidKey+immunize/6150&view=print. Accessed November 30, 2006.

29. The answer is b. Vaccines that contain live, attenuated viruses (yellow fever, oral polio, oral typhoid, and MMR vaccines) should not be given to immunocompromised patients. Inactivated polio is safe, as is the parenteral typhoid vaccine. Cholera immunization is no longer recommended for travelers.

Weller PF. Immunizations for travel. Available at http://www.utdol. com/utd/content/topic.do?topidKey+immunize/6150&view=print. Accessed November 30, 2006.

30. The answer is a. (*South-Paul, pp 211–220.*) In some patients COCs cause a small increase in blood pressure. This risk increases with age. Both estrogen and progestin are known to cause blood pressure elevations, so changing formulations of COC or using progestin-only pills may not lead to problem resolution. Once COCs are discontinued, blood pressure usually resolves within 3 months.

31. The answer is e. (*South-Paul, pp 211–220.*) Side effects of COCs include androgenic effects (hair growth, male pattern baldness, nausea.) and estrogenic effects (nausea, breast tenderness, and fluid retention). Weight gain is thought to be a common side effect, but multiple studies have failed to show it to be a statistically significant side effect. The side effect most frequently cited as the reason for stopping use of COCs is irregular bleeding. It is common in the first 3 months of use, and generally diminishes over time.

32. The answer is c. (*South-Paul, pp 211–220.*) The use of COC pills is associated with a threefold risk of venous thromboembolism. COCs have a protective effect against ovarian cancer and endometrial cancer. The risk of hemorrhagic stroke is not increased by the use of COCs, and they have not been shown in studies to impact carbohydrate metabolism in a statistically significant way.

33. The answer is e. (*South-Paul, pp 211–220.*) Progestin-only pills prevent conception through suppression of ovulation, thickening of cervical mucus, alteration of the endometrium, and inhibition of tubal transport. The effectiveness of this method is dependent on consistency of use. In fact, if a pill is taken even 3 hours late, an alternative form of contraception should be used for 48 hours. There is no hormone-free period with these pills, and they should be taken every day. The pills do not carry an increased risk for thromboembolism, and the World Health Organization has reported this form of contraception to be safe for women with a history of venous thrombosis, pulmonary embolism, diabetes, obesity, or hypertension. Nursing women can use this pill, but there is FDA approval for use in others as well. In general, progestin-only pills protect against ectopic pregnancy by lowering the chance of conception. However, if progestin-only pill users get pregnant, the chance of ectopic pregnancy is 6–10%, higher than the rate found in women not using contraception. Therefore, users should be aware of the symptoms for ectopic pregnancy.

34. The answer is d. (*South-Paul, pp 211–220.*) Oral contraceptive pills containing estrogen and progestin components are contraindicated in smokers over 35, due to an increased risk of thromboembolic events. An intravaginal ring or transdermal patch that releases estrogen and progestin are also contraindicated in smokers over 35 for the same reason. IUDs should not be used in women with more than one sexual partner, or in people whose partner has more than one partner. IUDs should not be used in people at high risk for developing a sexually transmitted infection, as women with an IUD are more likely to develop pelvic inflammatory disease after a sexually transmitted infection as compared with those using hormonal methods. An injectable long acting progestin would therefore be the best choice in this woman.

35. The answer is c. (*South-Paul, pp 211–220.*) Emergency contraception is appropriate when no contraception was used (including cases of sexual assault), or when there is contraceptive failure. They should be used within 72 hours of intercourse, well before implantation (implantation occurs 5–7 days after intercourse). ECPs involve limited hormonal exposure, and therefore have not been shown to increase the risk of venous thromboembolism, stroke or myocardial infarction. In fact, there are no medical contraindications to the use of emergency contraception pills. They do not disrupt an already implanted pregnancy and do not cause birth defects. Progestin ECPs prevent 85% of expected pregnancies when used correctly, and combined ECPs prevent 75% of expected pregnancies. They are not 100% effective in pregnancy prevention. There is no need to perform a pregnancy test when prescribing.

Doctor-Patient Issues

Questions

Communication

36. You are performing a medical interview with a patient and having some difficulty obtaining accurate information regarding the events that brought him into the office. Which of the following physician communication tactics leads to the collection of the most accurate information?

a. Controlling the interview with more directive questions
b. Using medical terms that the physician feels the patient can understand
c. Redirecting the patient if he/she strays from the relevant points
d. Involving the patient in his/her treatment plan
e. Using open-ended questions

37. You are seeing a 45-year-old woman who saw you 2 weeks ago because she felt fatigued. Her evaluation revealed previously undiagnosed type 2 diabetes, and she made today's appointment to discuss the next steps. She was on time for her 10:00 appointment, but because of a complicated patient, you didn't get into her room until 11:15. When you walk in, she appears extremely angry. How should you approach this situation?

a. Acknowledge her anger with a statement like, "You seem furious"
b. Be empathetic, understanding that her anger is likely displaced and a reaction to her new chronic illness
c. Explore the reasons for her anger if she brings it up
d. Explain the situation with a statement like, "My last patient was very complex, and he really needed my attention"
e. Help the patient understand that her anger should be directed at the illness, not at you

38. You are seeing a cantankerous 65-year-old with hypertension. You are concerned that he is not taking his blood pressure medications. Of the following, which is the most effective way to measure his compliance to the prescribed medical regimen?

a. Have him bring in his medications so that you may perform pill counts
b. Measure serum blood levels of his medications
c. Ask him if he is taking his medications
d. Look for a reduction in his blood pressure in subsequent visits
e. Ask him specific questions about his medication name, dosage, and administration times

39. You are seeing a 65-year-old woman who has smoked for 50 years. You want her to quit, and are considering different communication tactics to use in the discussion. Which of the following is likely to be the most powerful motivator?

a. Point out the positive results that can be expected if she complies with your advice. "By quitting, you'll significantly reduce your chances of developing lung cancer."
b. Point out the consequences of not following your advice. "If you don't quit, you might develop lung cancer."
c. Empathize. "I'll bet that quitting is extremely difficult."
d. Provide data. "Evidence shows that one in 20 patients who try can quit smoking cold turkey."
e. Ask about their experience with the illness that she is at risk for. "Do you know anyone who has ever suffered with emphysema?"

40. A 23-year-old man is following up to discuss the results of laboratory tests you did at his complete physical examination 1 week ago. His HIV screen was positive, and you need to tell him this news. Of the following, which is the most appropriate approach?

a. Begin the session by inquiring about his understanding of HIV
b. Help him prepare for the information by using a statement like, "I'm afraid I have some bad news for you"
c. Ensure you schedule enough time to discuss treatment goals and options
d. Make sure he brings a support person into the room before you disclose the test results
e. Offer hope by saying, "I'm sure there will be a cure for this disease soon"

41. You are seeing a 36-year-old woman with a complex medical condition. You have explored how she views the problem, you thoroughly understand her point of view, and you have acknowledged to the patient that you understand her point of view. Which of the following communication tactics best describes this approach?

a. Empathy
b. Sympathy
c. Collaboration
d. Therapeutic alliance
e. Patient centeredness

42. Regarding patient education and counseling, which of the following statements is true?

a. Patients commonly believe that physicians give them too much information
b. Patients usually understand and remember most information from their physician
c. Patients are more likely to make behavior changes if they are given several options for change from which to choose
d. Physician eye contact has not been shown to improve patient recall
e. Patients feel patronized when physicians repeat information or check for patient understanding

Cultural Competency and Health Disparities

43. You are treating a 61-year-old Chinese immigrant for fatigue. After evaluating the cause, you diagnose type 2 diabetes. She is reluctant to make the dietary changes necessary to help treat the condition, as much of her culturally based diet has a high glycemic index inappropriate for diabetes. What is the most culturally appropriate response?

a. Ask to involve her Americanized children in future communication to help encourage the changes
b. Since her culture believes that health is a balance between yin and yang, tell her that the dietary changes you suggest will restore this balance
c. Organize an appointment with the patient and a diabetes educator who can better take the time and explain the etiology and dietary regimen necessary for diabetes
d. Inquire as to the patient's concept of the etiology of diabetes and any treatments she would like to try
e. Use a Chinese interpreter to ensure your message is being heard appropriately

44. You are caring for a Spanish-speaking patient and working with an interpreter. Which of the following statements is true regarding the effective use of a medically trained interpreter?

a. Greet the patient in his/her language
b. Arrange seats in a triad, and speak slowly, facing the interpreter
c. Act as if the interpreter is not present, speaking to the patient normally
d. Use as many nonverbal gestures as possible
e. If you get an inconsistent response, repeat the same question over again

45. A physician is having difficulty interacting with a patient who is an immigrant from India. The patient is not complying with treatment plans for his hypertension. To improve this, which of the following is the most appropriate approach?

a. Speak with Indian colleagues to better understand the Indian culture
b. Refer the patient to a physician from the same cultural background as the patient
c. Study the Indian culture as it relates to illness and healing, and offer alternatives for treatment consistent with the cultural norms
d. Listen to the patient's perspective, express your treatment plan, and focus on similarities and differences
e. Examine the cultures beliefs of Indians and use the belief to convince the patient to comply with treatment

46. You are working at a medical office whose population includes a large proportion of Native American patients. Which of the following health issues has a higher prevalence in this population than in other American population groups?

a. Hypertension
b. Coronary artery disease
c. Suicide
d. Asthma
e. Tuberculosis

47. You are working in an office that provides care to a large population of homeless patients. Which is true about medical illnesses in homeless children as compared with other groups of children?

a. Homeless children are more likely to develop type 2 diabetes
b. Homeless children experience a higher number of ear infections
c. Homeless children are more likely to have chronic illness
d. Homeless children are more likely to have depression
e. Homeless children are more likely to have attention deficit disorders

48. The office where you are working cares for a large amount of uninsured patients. Which of the following population subgroups is more likely to be uninsured than other ethnic minority groups?

a. Hispanics
b. African Americans
c. Southeast Asians
d. Native Americans
e. Pacific Islanders

49. You are working in an office that serves a large uninsured population. Which of the following is true regarding this population as compared to the privately insured population?

a. This population has fewer chronic health conditions
b. This population has a lower mortality rate
c. This population has a better general health status
d. This population has a better mental health status
e. This population has a higher rate of chronic disease among children

50. You are evaluating health disparities in your community and using mortality rates as a measure of overall health. Of the following, which population subgroup in the United States has the lowest mortality rate at each age of the lifespan?

a. African Americans
b. Hispanic Americans
c. Native Americans
d. Asian Americans
e. Non-Hispanic whites

51. You are evaluating a Hispanic patient with multiple somatic complaints and suspect a mental health disorder. Which of the following is true regarding mental health disparities in the United States today?

a. Mental health disorders are diagnosed less frequently in minority populations than in non-Hispanic white patients
b. It is uncommon for minority groups to express mental health disorders via somatization
c. Minority patients are more likely to be misdiagnosed than nonminority counterparts
d. Minorities who maintain cultural practices and resist involvement in the dominant culture have better mental health
e. Culture is less of a factor in mental health than in other organic syndromes or illnesses

Ethics and Professionalism

52. You are taking care of a 62-year-old woman with a urinary tract infection. You prescribe trimethoprim-sulfamethoxazole (Bactrim) for her infection, but forget to ask about allergies. The next day, she returns with significant hives, asking if Bactrim contains "sulfa," something she is allergic to. Which of the following fundamental principles of medical professionalism has been violated?

a. The principle of primacy of patient welfare
b. The principle of patient autonomy
c. The principle of social justice
d. The principle of professional competence
e. The principle of honesty with patients

53. You are working with a physician who is treating a patient for hypertension. The patient has a documented allergy to angiotensin converting enzyme inhibitors, and you note that the physician is prescribing them. You assume that the physician knows best, and do not let the physician know of the potential mistake. What professional responsibility have you violated?

a. Commitment to honesty with patients
b. Commitment to professional competence
c. Commitment to maintaining appropriate patient relationships
d. Commitment to improving quality of care
e. Commitment to maintaining trust

54. You are working as a student in the emergency room. After a cardiac arrest and a prolonged attempt at resuscitation, a patient dies. The attending physician asks if you would like to gain experience by practicing intubations on the patient who has died. You feel that this relates to one of your professional responsibilities, to maintain clinical competence, and consider the offer. Which fundamental principle of professionalism and ethics would be violated if you do this?

a. The principle of patient welfare
b. The principle of patient autonomy
c. The principle of social justice
d. The principle of honesty with patients
e. The principle of maintaining trust

55. In the elevator, your senior resident says, "Before I forget, make sure you send Mr. Davis home on his usual HIV medications." You know that there are new medications that he could take, that might give him a better antiviral response. There are other people in the elevator. What professional responsibility has your senior resident violated?

a. Commitment to maintaining trust
b. Commitment to improving quality of care
c. Commitment to professional competence
d. Commitment to scientific knowledge
e. Commitment to patient confidentiality

56. One of your patients is 6 months pregnant, and is found to have a medical condition that, if left untreated, will be life-threatening to both her and the fetus. She believes that God will take care of her and the baby, and she refuses medical intervention offered to her. Which of the following best describes the principle of patient autonomy in this case?

a. She has no right to refuse the intervention, based on the fact that her decision is lethal to both her and her unborn infant
b. She has no right to refuse the intervention, based on the fact that her decision is lethal to her infant
c. She has the right to refuse the intervention regardless of the condition
d. She has the right to refuse the intervention, only if the father of her baby agrees
e. She has the right to refuse the intervention if she is found competent to make the decision

57. You are caring for a 55-year-old man who recently has complained of chest pain. His electrocardiogram is abnormal, and you feel he should have a cardiac catheterization. After explaining the risks and benefits to him, he refuses the intervention. Which of the following responses best demonstrates the tenets of professionalism in this case?

a. Respect the patient's choice and continue to explore his reasons for refusing treatment
b. Explain to him that you think he is making a bad decision, and try to convince him to change his mind
c. Consult the ethics committee of the hospital
d. Consult a psychiatrist to determine the patient's competency
e. Discharge the patient from your practice because of the poor doctor-patient relationship you have with him

58. You are caring for a 38-year-old man with metastatic cancer. He thoroughly understands his condition, and realizes that he has only a few months to live. He asks that you do not tell his wife about his prognosis, as "she won't be able to take it." The patient's wife sees you in the hallway and says, "tell me the truth . . . how is his condition?" Which of the following responses best reflects an ethically sound course of action?

a. Tell her the truth about the situation because she has a right to know
b. Tell her the truth because you have the legal obligation to do so
c. Consult the ethics committee to help you make the decision
d. Do not tell the patient's wife, but inform her that you will not tell her husband about the conversation you've just had
e. Do not tell the patient's wife, but make an effort to encourage an open dialogue between her and her husband

Complementary and Alternative Medicine

59. The practice where you are working cares for a wide variety of patients. Of the following, which subgroup is most likely to explore and use complementary and alternative medicine (CAM)?

a. Children
b. College students
c. Men
d. Women
e. The elderly

60. You are treating a 75-year-old Caucasian man with benign prostatic hyperplasia (BPH). He would like to consider an herbal medication to control his symptoms. Which of the following is the best option for this condition?

a. Ginkgo biloba
b. *Hypericum* (St. John's wort)
c. Saw palmetto
d. Garlic
e. Glucosamine

61. Traditional therapies have offered limited benefit to a 55-year-old woman who suffers from migraine headaches, and she asks you about alternative therapies. She currently takes 325 mg of enteric-coated aspirin a day, and paroxetine, 20 mg daily. Which of the following has the lowest risk of toxicity or harm?

a. St. John's wort
b. Megavitamins
c. Macrobiotic diet
d. Gingko biloba
e. Acupuncture

62. You know that many of your patients have tried complementary and alternative medicines (CAMs), but also know that patients may not reveal this to their physicians. What percentage of patients that use complementary and alternative medicine practices reveal this information to their conventionally trained physicians?

a. Less than 5%
b. Approximately 10%
c. Approximately 30%
d. Approximately 50%
e. More than 50%

63. Of those patients who use CAM, how many use it as their exclusive treatment modality?

a. Less than 5%
b. Approximately 10%
c. Approximately 30%
d. Approximately 50%
e. Most patients who use CAM practices use them exclusively

Palliative Care

64. After a prolonged fight with metastatic breast cancer, your patient decides to forego further attempts at curative treatment and focus on palliative care. She has tried nonsteroidal anti-inflammatory agents and acetaminophen for management of her chronic bone pain, but this has been ineffective. Which of the following would be the best initial pain management regimen?

a. Dexamethasone or another steroid to get the pain under control then scheduled nonsteroidal anti-inflammatory medications to maintain pain control
b. A fentanyl patch at the lowest dose that controls the pain
c. Five milligrams of immediate release morphine sulfate every 4 hours, with a dose every 2 hours as needed
d. Sustained release morphine sulfate, with immediate release morphine used for breakthrough pain
e. A patient-controlled analgesia device using opioids

65. Your patient has terminal cancer with a life expectancy of less than 3 months. You are managing her chronic cancer pain with morphine sulfate. She has been stable for weeks, but is requiring increasing amounts of opiates to maintain pain control. Which of the following statements is true regarding this situation?

a. The patient's disease is progressing and you should increase her medication dosage
b. The patient's disease is progressing and you should change medications
c. The patient is developing tolerance and you should increase her medication
d. The patient is developing tolerance and you should maintain the dosage of medication to avoid dependence
e. The patient is developing tolerance and you should slowly withdraw medication

66. You are caring for a 68-year-old man who, one month ago, developed a rash. The rash consisted of grouped vesicles on erythematous bases in a dermatomal pattern. You effectively treated the rash, but the patient complained of a persistent burning and itching pain in the same area as the rash. The pain is significant and keeps him from sleeping. What is the best approach for long-term pain management in this patient?

a. Nonsteroidal anti-inflammatory agents
b. Opiate analgesics
c. Steroids
d. Anticonvulsants
e. Selective serotonin reuptake inhibitors

67. You are caring for a 65-year-old man with lung cancer. He was diagnosed 4 months ago, and is not expected to live for more than 2 months. He is experiencing dyspnea. His chest x-ray shows progression of his cancer, and his pulse oximetry shows a room air oxygen saturation of 94%. Which of the following is most likely to relieve his symptoms?

a. Opioids
b. Nebulized morphine
c. Steroids
d. Benzodiazepines
e. Albuterol

68. You are caring for a 68-year-old man who has had colon cancer for 3 years. Therapies have been unsuccessful, and he has chosen palliative care only. He complains of excessive fatigue, feeling tired after minimal activity, and lacking energy to perform the activities of daily living. He denies depression, and feels he is handling his diagnosis well with the support of his family and friends. His laboratory evaluation is normal, except for mild anemia. Which of the following therapies would be most likely to help his symptoms?

a. Transfusion
b. Nutritional supplementation
c. Selective serotonin reuptake inhibitors
d. Sedative hypnotics
e. A psychostimulant like methylphenidate

69. You are treating a 60-year-old patient with end stage ovarian cancer. You are concerned that she may be developing depression. Which of the following would be the most reliable symptom of depression in this patient?

a. Loss of appetite
b. Fatigue
c. Insomnia
d. Sadness
e. Anhedonia

70. You are caring for a 39-year-old woman who is dying of breast cancer. Her family wonders how to recognize the symptoms of impending death. Which of the following is a reliable sign that death is near in this patient?

a. Delirium
b. Desire to communicate with loved ones
c. Limited attention span
d. Desire for favorite food
e. Increased attention to dates and time

71. You are making a home visit to a 68-year-old man with terminal cancer. His family says that his breathing seems to be labored. Upon evaluation, you know that this is the "death rattle" that often signals approaching death. Which of the following drugs would be most useful in controlling this symptom?

a. Atropine
b. Ketorolac
c. Lorazepam
d. Haloperidol
e. Thorazine

Gay, Lesbian, Bisexual, and Transgender Issues

72. A 19-year-old sexually active homosexual male asks you about his risk for hepatitis. He is currently asymptomatic and unsure of his immune status. Which of the following would you recommend?

a. Vaccination against Hepatitis A only
b. Vaccination against Hepatitis B only
c. Vaccine against Hepatitis C only
d. Vaccinations against both Hepatitis A and B
e. Vaccinations against both Hepatitis B and C

73. A 26-year-old homosexual man presents with blood on the toilet paper when wiping. Examination of the anal mucosa reveals this:

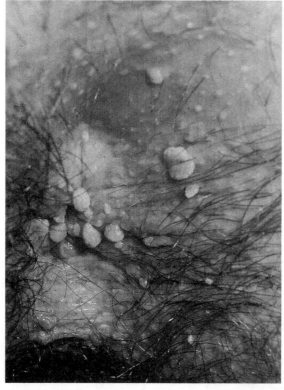

(Reproduced, with permission, from Wolff K, Johnson RA, Suurmond D. Fitzpatrick's Color Atlas and Synopsis of Clinical Dermatology, *5th ed. New York: McGraw-Hill, 2005: 891.)*

Which of the following statements is true regarding this condition?

a. This condition is rarely seen in men who are not immunocompromised
b. The patient's physician should consider anal cytologic screening with a Papinacolau (Pap) test
c. The patient should be treated with intramuscular penicillin once a week for 3 weeks
d. The patient should be treated with valciclovir
e. The patient should be treated with one dose of azithromycin

74. A 30-year-old gay male asks you about how his sexuality impacts his cancer risks. Which of the following statements most accurately reflect his risk for cancer?

a. Homosexual men have an increased rate of oral cancer
b. Homosexual men have an increased rate of colon cancer
c. Homosexual men have an increased rate of liver cancer
d. Homosexual men have an increased rate of testicular cancer
e. Homosexual men have an increased rate of anal cancer

75. You are caring for a 42-year-old lesbian woman. She has recently left a 10-year monogamous relationship, and is concerned about her risk for vaginal and other infections, once she resumes sexual activity with a new partner. Which of the following is true regarding her concern?

a. The rate of sexually transmitted infections (STIs) among lesbians is less than the rate in heterosexual women
b. The rate of genital warts is higher in lesbians than in heterosexual women
c. The rate of bacterial vaginosis is higher in lesbians than in heterosexual women
d. The rate of genital herpes is higher in lesbians than in heterosexual women
e. Sexually active lesbians have a lower prevalence of HIV than women who have sex exclusively with men

76. You are caring for a 40-year-old lesbian with no family history of breast cancer. She asks you about her risk of having breast cancer. Which of the following is true regarding breast cancer among lesbian women?

a. Breast cancer rates do not differ between lesbians and heterosexual women
b. Breast cancer rates are higher among lesbians because of nonparity
c. Breast cancer rates are higher among lesbians because of obesity
d. Breast cancer rates are higher among lesbians because of alcohol and tobacco use
e. Breast cancer rates are lower among lesbians because they generally use oral contraceptives less

77. You are caring for a 25-year-old lesbian. She asks you about Papinacolau (Pap) testing in lesbian women. Which of the following is true about cervical cancer screening in this population?

a. Lesbians do not need Pap testing
b. Lesbians do not need Pap testing, except if they are smokers
c. Lesbians need Pap testing, but less frequently than heterosexual women
d. Lesbians should be screened for cervical cancer at the same intervals that are recommended for heterosexual women
e. Lesbians should be screened for cervical cancer more frequently than heterosexual women

78. You are taking the complete history of a patient new to your office. The patient is dressed as a woman, but is biologically male. Further history reveals that the patient takes female hormones and is considering sexual reassignment surgery. What term best describes this person's condition?

a. Cross dresser
b. Bigender
c. Transvestite
d. Transsexual
e. Transgender

Doctor-Patient Issues

Answers

36. The answer is e. (*South-Paul, pp 663–668.*) Studies have shown that physicians often interrupt patients before they completely express their concerns. Physicians who do this and control the interview with directive questions often miss valuable and important information. These behaviors result in an incomplete clinical picture and a collection of inaccurate information. Information is also lost when physicians use medical jargon. Patients frequently believe they understand the jargon, but are often incorrect. Involving the patient in his/her treatment plan is important, but that does not lead to the collection of accurate information. The use of closed-ended questions limits the patients' ability to fully describe their concerns. Communication is enhanced and accuracy is improved when physicians use open-ended questions, allow patients to fully answer questions before interrupting, and avoid technical or medical jargon.

37. The answer is a. (*South-Paul, pp 663–668.*) Dealing with the angry patient is challenging for any health care provider. The natural reaction to anger is defensiveness, but a defensive response will often escalate the situation. The best approach is for the physician to first recognize the anger, then acknowledge it, try to understand it, and respond to it. If a physician senses that a patient is angry, but the patient has not volunteered this information, it is important to explore the anger. If the patient seems very upset, it may make him/her angrier if you minimize the situation by saying something like, "you seem a little upset." If a patient is extremely angry, choose words that seem to match the intensity of his/her feelings. In some instances anger is displaced, and may be truly directed at the disease process or illness. In that case, the appropriate response is empathy. However, in this setting, the anger is likely a response to the wait time that the patient has endured, and is less likely to be displaced. Placing the blame on your previous patient should be avoided, as it may make the current patient feel less important than the previous one.

38. The answer is e. (*South-Paul, pp 663–668.*) Compliance is a complex issue for physicians and patients. In patients who are noncompliant, the reasons usually relate to the patients' beliefs, goals and expectations. Asking the patient if he takes his medications is unlikely to yield accurate information, as the answer to this question is often an automatic "yes." However, patients will give accurate information about compliance about 80% of the time if the physician asks well-framed questions. By asking specific questions about names, dosages and times, the physician will be more likely to elicit information about compliance. Another tactic may be to give permission for admitting noncompliance by saying something like, "Some of my patients find it difficult to remember to take their medications. Does this ever happen to you?"

Performing pill counts, measuring serum blood levels and evaluating outcomes have not been shown in the medical literature to be effective measures of compliance.

39. The answer is a. (*South-Paul, pp 663–668.*) When motivating a patient to comply with a treatment regimen, it is important to explore their reasons for noncompliance. Once that is accomplished, the provider and patient should come to agreement on how to proceed. In this process, the physician can correct misconceptions, refer the patient to a trusted source of information, explore options or suggest alternatives. Fear is not an effective motivator in most cases. Therefore, pointing out consequences of not following advice, or bringing up images of suffering patients is not effective. While empathy is appropriate to enhance the doctor patient relationship, it is not always an effective motivational tool. Providing data often does not help, as patients do not see themselves as numbers and often do not understand how to apply the statistics to their situation. Patients are more likely to comply if you point out the positive results that can be expected by following your advice.

40. The answer is b. (*South-Paul, pp 663–668.*) When giving a patient bad news, attention should be given to the setting. Ensure the room is private and free of interruptions and that you have enough time for the visit. Some patients may want someone else present, but others may not. When suspicious that a test result may be positive, the physician may consider asking the patient in advance if they would like a support person present when reviewing the results. By beginning the session with an inquiry of the patient's knowledge, you are effectively giving the diagnosis without allowing the patient to prepare. Using a "warning" statement allows the patient to mentally prepare for the upcoming information. The discussion of treatment goals and options will likely overwhelm the patient, and should be deferred to a subsequent session. The physician should be hopeful, but realistic. Ensuring a cure for the disease may be detrimental.

41. The answer is a. *(South-Paul, pp 663–668.)* Empathy involves the three components described in the question. Sympathy does not require acknowledgement of understanding. Collaboration refers to the doctor and patient working together in treatment plans, as does a therapeutic alliance. Patient-centeredness involves understanding the patient, the illness or disease, its impact on his/her life, and the community to which the patient will look for relief and treatment.

42. The answer is c. *(South-Paul, pp 663–668.)* Patients commonly believe their physician does not give them enough information. However, studies show that patients often misunderstand or do not remember the information that physicians give them. Techniques physicians can employ to improve recall include simplification, repetition, giving specific information, and checking for understanding. Patients generally appreciate this, and generally do not feel this is patronizing. Nonverbal techniques including decreased interpersonal distance, more eye contact, and leaning toward the patient have been shown to improve recall. Patients are more likely to make behavior change if presented with several choices. However, too many options may be overwhelming. Statements like, "Your options are . . . " and "Which option do you think will be best for you?" are often helpful.

43. The answer is d. *(South-Paul, pp 669–679.)* Health, illness, and treatment is strongly influenced by cultural contexts. Although those trained in the United States have illness and treatment concepts based on biomedicine, many in other cultures define illness in other ways with different disease classifications and responses to them. Asking a patient of another culture what she thinks may be causing the problem and about treatment options demonstrates respect for the patient and her culture. Having Americanized relatives try to convince her would not respect her cultural beliefs. Pretending to understand her cultural and health beliefs may cause resentment. Continuing to focus on the biomedical model does not respect the cultural aspects of disease. Using an interpreter, while often necessary, does not address the underlying cultural issue.

44. The answer is a. *(South-Paul, pp 669–679.)* Recommendations for working with a medically trained interpreter include:

- Greet the patient in his/her own language if possible.
- Introduce yourself to everyone present.
- Arrange the seats in a triad, and address the patient.
- Speak clearly, in a normal voice volume.
- Use common terms and simple language structure.
- Express one idea at a time and pause for the interpreter.
- Expect the interpreter to use first person singular, verbatim translation
- Consider multiple meanings to nonverbal gestures.
- Ask the same questions in different ways if you get inconsistent or unconnected responses.
- Ask the interpreter to explain, but do not place the interpreter in the middle of conflicts.

45. The answer is d. *(South-Paul, pp 669–679.)* It is important to remember that physicians tend to focus on the biological process of disease, while patients focus on the illness experience, regardless of culture. Physicians should be familiar with the medically related cultural norms of the patients residing in their community, but also need to recognize that the norms are not stereotypical statements about all people from that culture. Individuals within groups may have different practices. As such, the most appropriate approach would be to Listen to your patient's perspective, Explain your plan, Acknowledge similarities and differences, Recommend an action and Negotiate a plan (LEARN).

46. The answer is c. *(South-Paul, pp 680–687.)* In the 2000 census, Native Americans made up only 0.7% of the population, but the prevalence of diabetes, obesity, alcoholism and suicide is substantially higher in this population than others.

47. The answer is b. *(South-Paul, pp 680–687.)* Homelessness results in poor health status and high service use among children. Homeless children experience a higher number of acute illness symptoms, including fever, ear infections, diarrhea, and asthma exacerbations. Unfortunately, the emergency department tends to be a primary source of care for this group, and visits are higher among this population.

48. The answer is a. *(South-Paul, pp 680–687.)* One-third of all nonelderly Hispanics living in the United States do not have health insurance.

Hispanics are more likely to be uninsured and are the fastest growing minority group in the United States. This makes it likely that the total number of uninsured people in the United States will increase.

49. The answer is a. (*South-Paul, pp 680–687.*) Interestingly, the uninsured have lower rates of chronic health conditions as compared with the insured population. The reason for his may reflect the fact that uninsured people often work in physically demanding jobs with fewer benefits. Those with chronic debilitating disease are unable to continue working and may go on public assistance. The uninsured have a higher mortality rate, poorer general health status and poorer mental health status. Uninsured children have similar rates of chronic disease and limitations of activity when compared with insured children.

50. The answer is d. (*South-Paul, pp 680–687.*) At each age of the lifespan African Americans, Hispanics, and Native Americans have a higher mortality rate than whites. Only Asians, in aggregate, average lower mortality rates than whites.

51. The answer is c. (*South-Paul, pp 680–687.*) Mental health disparities have existed in minority cultures for decades. The practice of psychiatry is heavily influenced by culture, perceptions of illness and appropriate treatment. Mental health disorders are diagnosed more commonly in non-whites than in their white counterparts. This may be partly due to poor validation of the DSM IV and the unfamiliarity of many psychiatrists with culturally defined syndromes and folk healing systems. Screening is difficult because there is a lack of language-specific validated instruments, and interpreters may miss nuances in translation. This leads to misdiagnosis. Many cultures express distress as somatic complaints. It is well-known that feeling accepted in society, increased acculturation and a good transition to the new culture decreases mental health issues, while increased resistance to new culture lowers mental health.

52. The answer is a. (*Brennan, pp 243–246.*) There are three fundamental principles of professionalism. The first is the principle of primacy of patient welfare. This is based on a dedication to serving the interest of the patient, and deals with doing no harm. This is the principle violated in the question. The principle of patient autonomy involves empowering patients to make informed decisions regarding their treatment. The principle of social justice involves working to eliminate discrimination in health care. Professional competence is a professional responsibility, not a fundamental principle, and deals with commitment to lifelong learning and maintaining medical knowledge. Patient honesty is also a responsibility, and deals with informed consent and acknowledging medical errors.

53. The answer is d. *(Brennan, pp 243–246.)* Improving quality of care is a professional responsibility that all physicians must embrace. The commitment involves maintaining clinical competence, but also working collaboratively with other professionals to reduce medical error. Honesty deals with informed consent and acknowledging errors with patients. Maintaining appropriate relationships deals with not exploiting patient relationships. Commitment to maintaining trust involves managing conflict of interests.

54. The answer is b. *(Brennan, pp 243–246.)* Fundamental principles of professionalism (patient welfare, patient autonomy, and social justice) are central to the job of being a physician. Despite the fact that the patient would not be harmed if the student practiced the procedure, the patient was not given the chance to make an informed decision about participating in this activity. Therefore, autonomy has been violated.

55. The answer is e. *(Brennan, pp 243–246.)* When other people can hear, it is important to ensure patient confidentiality. Appropriate safeguards should be applied to the disclosure of any patient information, including sensitive information regarding diagnosis and treatment. Despite the fact that the patient may do better on the new regimen, it is not appropriate to discuss it in the presence of others not associated with the patient's case.

56. The answer is e. *(Brennan, pp 243–246.)* The principle of patient autonomy requires physicians to be honest with their patients about treatment options, as well as the options if treatment is refused. Patient's decisions about their care are paramount, as long as those decisions are made competently. However, in difficult cases such as this one, it is recommended that legal counsel be obtained.

57. The answer is a. *(Brennan, pp 243–246.)* Convincing a patient to change his mind disregards patient autonomy. Consulting an ethics committee and evaluating the patient's competency are unnecessary at this point. Discharging the patient from your practice for disagreeing with you would be inappropriate.

58. The answer is e. *(Brennan, pp 243–246.)* Patient confidentiality demands that you maintain safeguards related to the disclosure of patient information. This is dictated by the patient, even if the wife is the other person in the communication triad.

59. The answer is d. *(South-Paul, pp 698–706.)* Rates of CAM use are significant in all populations, but studies have shown that women are consistently more likely to explore and use CAM. Women are frequently central to the health care decisions made in a family, and when surveyed, 49% of women have used CAM. Other surveys have shown that 50% of patients with cancer or HIV will use unconventional medical practices at some point during their illness. CAM is gaining public interest, and becoming increasingly popular in the United States.

60. The answer is c. *(South-Paul, pp 698–706.)* Systematic reviews of controlled trials have shown that saw palmetto is as effective as finasteride in relieving symptoms of BPH. However, its use did not result in a decreased prostate volume. Gingko biloba has been studied in people with dementia, and garlic has been studied in people with heart disease. A number of placebo-controlled trials have shown that St. John's wort may be effective in the treatment of depression. Glucosamine is a natural medicine that is primarily used to help arthritis symptoms.

61. The answer is e. *(South-Paul, pp 698–706.)* When discussing complementary and alternative medicine, physicians should help patients make informed choices. Many practices, including acupuncture, biofeedback, homeopathy, and meditation are low risk if used by competent practitioners. Many herbal substances can interact with traditional medications and cause harm. St. John's wort can cause serotonin syndrome when used with a selective serotonin reuptake inhibitor like paroxetine. Megavitamins carry with them the risk of toxicity. Special diets, including the macrobiotic diet (high complex carbohydrate, low fat, vegetarian diet) may have harmful effects, including undesirable changes in weight and bowel habits. Gingko biloba has antiplatelet effects, and may cause bleeding when taken with aspirin.

62. The answer is c. (*South-Paul, pp 698–706.*) There is a major communication gap between physicians and the public regarding CAM practices. More than 70% of patients that use CAM do not reveal this to their conventional physicians. Often, they fear reprisal from their physician. If physicians are open to hearing about therapies, and react to the knowledge in a nonjudgmental fashion, patients will feel more comfortable sharing the information, and patient care will be improved.

63. The answer is a. (*South-Paul, pp 698–706.*) The overwhelming majority of patients who use CAM use it as an adjunct to more traditional western therapies. Less than 5% use CAM exclusively. In general, patients who use CAM do not harbor an "antiscience" sentiment. Patients who use CAM do not include a disproportionate number of uneducated, poor or mentally ill representatives. Often, the attraction to CAM is philosophical, and is consistent with the patient's overall health beliefs.

64. The answer is c. (*South-Paul, pp 714–729.*) The World Health Organization published guidelines for pain control in 1996. These guidelines have been well-studied and lead to effective pain control in most situations. In general, failing nonopioid pain control should lead to the use of opioid analgesics. Steroids have limited, if any, use in chronic cancer pain. Fentanyl patches, even at the lowest dose, may be excessive in opiate naïve patients, and should never be used alone. Most start with immediate release morphine sulfate to determine a baseline need. This can be converted to sustained release quickly, and titrated based on pain control. Patient-controlled analgesia devices have an important role, but require intravenous or subcutaneous administration, and should not be used first-line, unless pain is extreme.

65. The answer is a. (*South-Paul, pp 714–729.*) Managing chronic cancer pain with opiates is often concerning for physicians. Many fear addiction and are concerned about causing harm. It is important to remember that there is no specific limit to opioid dose, and medications should be titrated to pain control or development of significant side effects. Fear of addiction should not hinder the use of opiates in this situation. Addiction is a rare occurrence in patients with terminal illness, especially in patients without a history of drug abuse. In patients on previously steady doses, dose escalation generally means the disease is progressing rather than tolerance. Tolerance, like addiction, is rarely seen.

66. The answer is d. (*South-Paul, pp 714–729.*) Neuropathic pain, like that described from shingles in this question, frequently requires opioids in the short term, but often requires the use of other medications for long-term relief. Commonly used medications includes tricyclic antidepressants, anticonvulsants (valproic acid, carbamazepine, gabapentin are the most common), and antihistamines. The data on using selective serotonin reuptake inhibitors are unconvincing.

67. The answer is a. (*South-Paul, pp 714–729.*) Dyspnea, like pain, is a subjective sensation. It can be present in the absence of hypoxia. Opioids can relieve breathlessness associated with advanced cancer by an unclear mechanism. Nebulized morphine isn't more effective than placebo. Steroids and albuterol are useful for dyspnea caused by bronchospasm, but that is unlikely in this case. Anxiolytics, like benzodiazepines and buspirone, may help if anxiety is a significant component, but that is usually expressed by patients as a feeling of "choking" or "suffocation."

68. The answer is e. (*South-Paul, pp 714–729.*) Excessive fatigue seen with end-stage cancer may result from direct tumor effects, paraneoplastic neuropathy, or tumor involvement of the CNS. It is often an effect of therapy. When no specific cause is apparent, as in this question, therapy is difficult. Transfusion is unlikely to be beneficial given his hemoglobin level. There is no evidence that the patient has a nutritional deficit, and supplementation may not be helpful. Although fatigue is frequently seen as a symptom of depression and may respond to selective serotonin reuptake inhibitor therapy, in this case it is unlikely. Sleeping pills would not help unless insomnia is the cause. A short course of steroids or a psychostimulant can increase energy and improve mood.

69. The answer is e. (*South-Paul, pp 714–729.*) It is commonly assumed that all patients with cancer are, and should be, depressed. Physicians often do not recognize depression because they feel they would be depressed in the same situation. While neurovegetative symptoms are a compelling indication of depression in the physically healthy patient, they may be less reliable for the diagnosis of depression in patients with advanced cancer. Loss of appetite may be due to therapy, fatigue may be due to insomnia from untreated pain. Sadness may be appropriate, given the diagnosis. Anhedonia is a useful, if not the most useful symptom to monitor. Also helpful are hopelessness, guilt, and a wish to die.

70. The answer is c. (*South-Paul, pp 714–729.*) As death approaches, there are several signs that portend its arrival. Delirium may be a result of medication, and by itself is not a good indicator. Other indicators are:

- Remaining bedbound
- Confusion
- Cool and mottled extremities
- The "death rattle"
- Decreased hearing/vision
- Difficulty swallowing
- Decreased conversation
- Decreased oral intake
- Disorientation to time
- Drowsiness progressing to somnolence for extended periods
- Dry mouth
- Hallucinations
- Increased distance from all but a few intimate others
- Decreased attention span
- Profound weakness

71. The answer is a. (*South-Paul, pp 714–729.*) Atropine can decrease secretions and help the "death rattle." Other medications that may be useful include scopolamine, glycopyrolate, mycosamine, or morphine. Ketorolac may help pain, lorazepam may help restlessness, haloperidol and thorazine may help agitation and hallucinations, both of which are also symptoms of impending death.

72. The answer is d. (*South-Paul, pp 688–697.*) The unique health needs of gay men may often be overlooked by physicians, especially if not alert to appropriate and sympathetic sexual history-taking. Since Hepatitis A is transmitted orally/fecally, and many gay men participate in oral/anal sexual activity, vaccination against Hepatitis A is appropriate. Since hepatitis B is transmitted through blood and body fluids, and sometimes by anal intercourse, Hepatitis B vaccination is indicated. There is no vaccination against Hepatitis C.

73. The answer is b. (*South-Paul, pp 688–697.*) The picture above represents infection with Human Papilloma Virus (HPV). The prevalence of this infection is high, and in one study, 65.9% of HIV negative gay men were found to be positive for anal HPV. Penicillin treats syphilis, valciclovir treats herpes and azithromycin treats Chlamydia and gonorrhea (high doses of azithromycin are needed to treat gonorrhea than Chlamydia). Men infected with HPV have been shown to have anal dysplasia, and cytologic screening should be considered for gay men positive for HPV.

74. The answer is e. *(South-Paul, pp 688–697.)* The increase in anal cancer in homosexual men is due to the increase in anal HPV infection seen in the gay male population. This is even seen in men without HIV. The other cancers listed do not seem to have an increased incidence in gay men.

75. The answer is c. *(South-Paul, pp 688–697.)* Generally, lesbians are felt to be at less risk for STIs than heterosexual women. However, most studies indicate comparable rates of STIs between lesbians and heterosexual women. Interestingly, the type of STI is different. Genital warts and genital herpes are more common in heterosexuals, with bacterial vaginosis being more common in lesbians. There is a mistaken belief that lesbians are not at risk for acquiring HIV. However, it has been shown that sexually active lesbians have a *higher* prevalence of HIV than women who have sex exclusively with men.

76. The answer is a. *(South-Paul, pp 688–697.)* Survey data from almost 12,000 women found no difference in breast cancer rates between lesbians and heterosexual women. Intuitively, one would think cancer rates would be higher because of nulliparity and higher rates of obesity. However, well-designed prospective studies have not been done to establish that as fact.

77. The answer is d. *(South-Paul, pp 688–697.)* Cervical cancer may be less prevalent in women who have never had heterosexual vaginal intercourse, however even in women reporting that they have never had sex with a man, up to 20% were found to have HPV DNA. Also, many physicians assume self-reported lesbians to have never had sex with a man, when some studies have reported that up to 79% of lesbians have reported having sex with a male in the past. Therefore, physicians should follow Pap smear screening guidelines in place for all women regardless of the woman's reported sexuality.

78. The answer is d. *(South-Paul, pp 688–697.)* Transgender is an umbrella term describing a group of people who cross culturally defined gender categories. Cross dressers wear the clothes of the other gender, but may not completely identify with that gender. Bigender individuals identify with both genders. Transvestites dress as another gender, but have not considered surgery. Transexuals wish to change their sex, and have considered or undertaken surgery.

Biostatistics

Questions

Biostatistics

79. You note that in your practice, a large number of women with a family history of breast cancer in a first degree relative develop breast cancer themselves. You evaluate a number of charts, and find that 5% of the women in your practice who have breast cancer have a family history, but only 2% of women without breast cancer have a family history. Given this information, what is the sensitivity of using family history as a predictor of breast cancer in your patient population?

a. 2%
b. 5%
c. 93%
d. 95%
e. 98%

80. You are reading a population study that reports 90% of people with lung cancer are smokers. Thirty percent of the people without lung cancer are also smokers. Given this information, what is the specificity using smoking as a predictor of lung cancer?

a. 10%
b. 30%
c. 40%
d. 70%
e. 90%

81. You are determining whether or not to use a rapid streptococcal antigen test to screen for streptococcal pharyngitis. You find that that 2% of people with strep throat actually test negative using this test. Of the following, which statement best describes this situation?

a. The sensitivity of the test is 2%
b. The specificity of the test is 98%
c. The test has a 2% false negative rate
d. The test has a 2% false positive rate
e. The test has a positive predictive value of 98%

82. You are reading a medical journal and come across an article about diabetes. The study followed 10,000 patients over 3 years. At the start of the study, 2000 people had diabetes. At the end of the study, 1000 additional people developed diabetes. What was the incidence of diabetes during the study?

a. 10%
b. 12.5%
c. 20%
d. 30%
e. 50%

83. You are reading a study that compares cholesterol levels in children whose fathers died from a myocardial infarction with cholesterol levels in children whose fathers died from other causes. The p value obtained in the test was <0.001. What does this value indicate?

a. There was no difference in cholesterol levels between the two groups
b. The difference in the cholesterol levels was less than 0.1%
c. There is a less than 0.1% probability that the results obtained in this study were incorrect
d. There is a less than 0.1% probability that the results obtained in this study occurred because of a sampling error
e. If the null hypothesis is true, there is a less than 0.1% probability of obtaining a test statistic equal to or more extreme than the one obtained

84. You are considering using a new influenza screening test. You find a study that evaluated 1000 patients with this new test. Of these 1000 patients, 400 had the disease. 300 of those had positive tests, and 100 of those had a negative test. Of the 600 that did not have the disease, 200 had positive tests, and 400 had negative tests. What is the positive predictive value of this test?

a. 50%
b. 60%
c. 66%
d. 75%
e. 80%

85. You find that many of your patients that have gone to the emergency department with chest pain have a negative set of initial cardiac enzymes. Most of those with a negative set of initial enzymes did not have a heart attack. You decide to evaluate 100 of your patients who have gone to the emergency department with chest pain to find out if an initial set of negative enzymes by itself is a good predictor of those that are not having a myocardial infarction (MI). Of those 100 patients, 20 of them had acute MIs. Of those 20, 10 had a positive set of enzymes initially. Of the 80 that did not have an acute MI, none of them had a positive set of initial enzymes. Given this information, what is the negative predictive value of the initial set of cardiac enzymes in your patient population?

a. 20%
b. 22%
c. 50%
d. 89%
e. 100%

Biostatistics

Answers

79. The answer is b. *(Rosner, pp 45–66.)* Sensitivity is thought of as the probability that a symptom is present given that the person has the disease. In the above example, the "symptom" in question is a family history of breast cancer. Of women that have breast cancer, 5% have a family history; therefore the sensitivity of using family history as a predictor of breast cancer is 5%.

80. The answer is d. *(Rosner, pp 45–66.)* Specificity can be thought of as the probability that the symptom is *not* present given that a person does not have a disease. In the above example, the "symptom" is smoking. Of people that do not have lung cancer, 30% of them are smokers, indicating that 70% of them are not smokers. Of the people who do not have lung cancer, 70% of them do not smoke.

81. The answer is c. *(Rosner, pp 45–66.)* A false negative is defined as a person who tests negative, but who is actually positive. In the above example, 2% of the positive people test negative. Therefore, the false negative rate is 2% in this case. Sensitivity is defined as the probability that the test would be positive, given that the person has strep throat. The specificity is the probability that the test would be negative if the person does *not* have strep. The false positive rate is defined as the percent of people who test positive, but are actually negative. The positive predictive value is the probability that a person has an illness, given that the test is positive.

82. The answer is b. *(Rosner, pp 45–66.)* The incidence of a disease is the probability that a person with no prior disease will develop a new case of the disease over a specific time period. In this case, 1000 people developed diabetes. In the study, only 8000 people began with no prior disease. Therefore, the incidence is 1000/8000 or 12.5%. The prevalence is the probability of having a disease at a specific point in time, and is obtained by dividing the number of people with the disease by the number of people in the study.

83. The answer is e. *(Rosner, pp 273–312.)* The p value for any hypothesis test is the level at which we would be indifferent between accepting or rejecting the null hypothesis given the sample data at hand. It can also be thought of as the probability of obtaining a test statistic as extreme or more extreme than the actual test statistic obtained, given that the null hypothesis is true. It does not reflect the absolute difference in the data between groups, and does not reflect the *correctness* of the data in the sample.

84. The answer is b. The positive predictive value refers to the probability that a positive test correctly identifies an individual that actually has the disease. Using a 4 × 4 chart:

	Disease present	Disease absent	Total
Test positive	A = 300	B = 200	500
Test negative	C = 100	D = 400	500
Total	400	600	**1000**
Positive predictive value = A/(A+B), or 300/500 = 60%			

Mahutte NG, Duleba AJ. Evaluating Diagnostic Tests. http://www.utdol.com/utd/content/topic.do?topicKey=genr_med/28312&type=A&selectedTitle=1~5, accessed 12/6/2006

85. The answer is d. The negative predictive value is the probability that a negative test correctly identifies an individual who does not have the disease. Using a 4 × 4 chart:

	Disease present	Disease absent	Total
Test positive	A = 10	B = 0	10
Test negative	C = 10	D = 80	90
Total	20	80	**100**
Negative predictive value = D/(C+D), or 80/90 = 89%			

Mahutte NG, Duleba AJ. Evaluating Diagnostic Tests. http://www.utdol.com/utd/content/topic.do?topicKey=genr_med/28312&type=A&selectedTitle=1~5, accessed 12/6/2006

Acute Complaints

Questions

86. You are evaluating a 36-year-old man in your office with the chief complaint of abdominal pain. Which of the following characteristics of the pain, if present, would lead you toward an emergent evaluation?

a. The pain is located in the right lower quadrant
b. The pain began suddenly
c. The pain is described as a "gnawing" sensation
d. The pain is worse after eating
e. The pain is associated with emesis

87. A 42-year-old woman presents to your office complaining of abdominal pain. She describes upper abdominal pain that radiates to her scapula. For which of the following is this description classic?

a. Acute appendicitis
b. Pancreatitis
c. Gallbladder disease
d. Esophageal spasm
e. Gastroesophageal reflux disease

88. An 80-year-old man presents with mild, crampy, bilateral lower quadrant pain, decreased appetite, and low-grade fever for about 48 hours. Which of the following is most likely?

a. Small bowel obstruction
b. Appendicitis
c. Constipation
d. Irritable bowel syndrome
e. Pancreatitis

89. While performing an abdominal examination on a 42-year-old woman in your office, she suddenly stops inspiratory effort during deep palpation of the right upper quadrant. Which of the following problems is this most suggestive of?

a. Hepatitis
b. Gallstones
c. Cholecystitis
d. Pancreatitis
e. Right-sided renal calculi

90. You are evaluating a 64-year-old man with abdominal pain. Your differential diagnosis includes diverticulitis, perforated diverticuli, and appendicitis. What imaging study would be most helpful to establish the diagnosis?

a. Abdominal radiograph
b. Ultrasound of the abdomen and pelvis
c. Computed tomography (CT) scan of the abdomen and pelvis
d. Magnetic resonance imaging (MRI) of the abdomen and pelvis
e. Colonoscopy

91. A 67-year-old presents to your office with a complaint of gnawing abdominal pain in the epigastrum and a sensation of hunger. She has a 50-pack-year history of tobacco use, and notes that her stool has become darker within the last 2 weeks. Which of the following is the most likely cause of her illness?

a. *Helicobacter pylori* infection
b. Nonsteroidal anti-inflammatory drug (NSAID) abuse
c. Alcoholism
d. Gallstones
e. Gastroparesis

92. A 26-year-old man presents with 3 months of heartburn. He also complains of regurgitation, belching, and occasional dry cough. His symptoms are worse when he is lying down. He denies melena, weight loss, or dysphagia. What is the appropriate next step, if you suspect gastroesophageal reflux disease (GERD) in this patient?

a. Treat with H2 receptor antagonists, a proton pump inhibitor or a prokinetic agent and evaluate the response
b. Obtain a barium swallow

c. Obtain a CT scan of the abdomen with oral and IV contrast
d. Obtain an ultrasound of the abdomen
e. Perform an esophagogastroduodenoscopy (EGD)

93. A 44-year-old woman is admitted to the hospital for acute right upper quadrant pain for 4 hours consistent with biliary colic, fever, and a positive Murphy's sign. She has a history of asymptomatic gallstones, identified incidentally several years ago. Her laboratory evaluation is as follows:

WBC:	17.5 K/uL (H) with a left shift
Aspartate aminotransferase AST:	88 U/L (H)
Alanine aminotransferase (ALT):	110 U/L (H)
Alkaline Phosphatase:	330 U/L (H)
Bilirubin (total):	3.2 mg/dL (H)

What would the next test of choice be?
a. Ultrasound of the abdomen
b. CT scan of the abdomen
c. MRI of the abdomen
d. Endoscopic retrograde cholangiopancreatography (ERCP)
e. Cholescintigraphy (HIDA or PISIDA)

94. You have diagnosed a patient with acute pancreatitis. What is the most common cause of this condition?

a. Gallstones
b. Alcohol abuse
c. Iatrogenic
d. Idiopathic
e. Hyperlipidemia

95. You are concerned about panreatitis in a 44-year-old woman with acute symptoms. Which of the following laboratory tests is most specific for pancreatitis?

a. White blood cell count
b. Amylase
c. Lipase
d. AST
e. ALT

96. You are seeing a 53-year-old man who was hospitalized for pancreatitis. His admission laboratory studies include a white blood cell count of 18,000/mm³, glucose of 153 mg/dL, lactate dehydrogenase of 254 IU/L, and AST of 165 U/L. According to Ranson's criteria, which of these factors suggest a poor prognosis in this patient?

a. Age
b. White blood cell count
c. Glucose
d. LDH
e. AST

97. A 22-year-old Caucasian female college student complains of diffuse lower abdominal pain. It has been present for approximately 5 months and gets better with defecating. The onset is associated with more frequent and loose bowel movements (three to five times per day). Sometimes the diarrhea is watery with mucus, but she denies blood or bloating. There has been no weight loss, and no nighttime symptoms. What is the most likely diagnosis?

a. Ulcerative colitis
b. Irritable bowel syndrome
c. Crohn's disease
d. Lactose intolerance
e. Diverticulitis

98. A 65-year-old man presents to you complaining of abdominal pain. His pain is associated with anorexia, bloating, nausea and vomiting. He is afebrile and denies fever. On examination, his abdomen appears distended, and he has absent bowel sounds. Abdominal percussion produces tympani. What would his abdominal x-ray likely show?

a. A fecalith in the right lower quadrant
b. Free intraperitoneal air
c. Stool throughout the colon
d. Proximally dilated loops of bowel
e. Stones in the right upper quadrant

99. You are caring for a 26-year-old generally healthy woman. She is sexually active and currently in a monogamous relationship. You recently completed her annual examination. Her Pap smear reports "atypical squamous cells of undetermined significance." Human papillomavirus testing was negative. Which of the following is the most appropriate next step?

a. Repeat the Pap smear immediately
b. Treat the patient with metronidazole and repeat the Pap smear when the course of antibiotics is finished
c. Repeat the Pap smear in 4–6 months
d. Repeat the Pap smear in 1 year
e. Perform colposcopy

100. You are caring for a 24-year-old generally healthy woman. She is sexually active and currently in a monogamous relationship, using oral contraceptives. You recently completed her annual examination. Her Pap smear reports "atypical squamous cells of undetermined significance." Human papillomavirus testing was positive. Which of the following is the most appropriate next step?

a. Repeat the Pap smear immediately
b. Repeat the Pap smear in 4–6 months
c. Repeat the Pap smear in 1 year
d. Perform colposcopy
e. Treat the patient with imiquimod (Aldara) and repeat the Pap smear after the treatment is complete

101. You are caring for a 40-year-old obese woman with mild hypertension. She is sexually active with her husband of 16 years, and had a tubal ligation after her son was born 5 years ago. One year ago, her Pap smear reported "atypical squamous cells of undetermined significance." Human papillomavirus testing at your institution was unavailable. You repeated the Pap smear at 4 months and 8 months after the initial sample was taken. Both of those samples were normal. Which of the following is the most appropriate next step?

a. Repeat the Pap smear immediately
b. Repeat the Pap smear in 4–6 months
c. Repeat the Pap smear in 1 year
d. Perform colposcopy
e. Treat the patient with fluconazole (Diflucan) and repeat the Pap smear after the treatment is complete

102. You are caring for a 28-year-old generally healthy woman. She is currently not sexually active, but has had multiple partners in the past. You recently completed her annual examination. Her Pap smear reports "atypical squamous cells of undetermined significance, favor low-grade squamous intraepithelial lesion." Which of the following is the most appropriate next step?

a. Repeat the Pap smear immediately
b. Repeat the Pap smear in 4–6 months
c. Repeat the Pap smear in 1 year
d. Perform colposcopy
e. Perform endometrial biopsy

103. You are caring for a 34-year-old generally healthy woman. She is sexually active and currently in a monogamous relationship with her husband, using oral contraceptives. You recently completed her annual examination. Her Pap smear reports "atypical glandular cells," but does not specify if those cells are endocervical or endometrial in origin. She has not had any abnormal vaginal bleeding. Which of the following is the most appropriate next step?

a. Repeat the Pap smear immediately
b. Repeat the Pap smear in 4–6 months
c. Repeat the Pap smear in 1 year
d. Perform colposcopy
e. Perform endometrial biopsy

104. You are caring for a 46-year-old generally healthy woman. She is sexually active with her husband only. You recently completed her annual examination. Her Pap smear reports "atypical glandular cells" and are reported to be of endometrial origin. She does not report any abnormal vaginal bleeding. Which of the following is the most appropriate next step?

a. Repeat the Pap smear immediately
b. Repeat the Pap smear in 4–6 months
c. Repeat the Pap smear in 1 year
d. Perform colposcopy
e. Perform endometrial biopsy

105. A 21-year-old woman is being evaluated for fatigue. Further history reveals weakness, exercise intolerance and a craving for chewing ice that has occurred over the last few weeks. Laboratory analysis reveals a hemoglobin of 8.7 g/dL. What is the likely cause of her anemia?

a. Lead
b. Iron deficiency
c. Chronic disease
d. Vitamin B-12 deficiency
e. Folic acid deficiency

106. A 20-year-old woman has had menorrhagia leading to anemia. Which of the following regimens would lead to the most iron being absorbed?

a. 300 mg iron sulfate twice a day
b. 300 mg iron sulfate with ascorbic acid twice a day
c. 300 mg iron sulfate with calcium carbonate twice a day
d. 300 mg iron gluconate twice a day
e. 300 mg iron gluconate with calcium carbonate twice a day

107. A 60-year-old man is being evaluated for fatigue, weakness, and exercise intolerance. Laboratory assessment reveals:

Hemoglobin 9.1 mg/dL (L)
Serum iron 46 mcg/dL (L)
Ferritin 9 ng/mL (L)
Total iron binding capacity (TIBC) 626 mcg/dL (H)
Mean corpuscular volume (MCV) 76 fL (L)

What is the most common cause of this condition?

a. Blood loss
b. Poor nutrition
c. Inadequate absorption of iron
d. Chronic disease
e. Folic acid deficiency

108. You are caring for a 64-year-old woman with longstanding type 2 diabetes mellitus. She comes to you complaining of fatigue. Screening laboratory analysis reveals a glycosolated hemoglobin level of 9.8%. Her hemoglobin is 10.4 g/dL, and her mean corpuscular volume is 76 fL (L). Further laboratory analysis reveals a serum iron of 40 mcg/dL (L), a total iron binding capacity of 188 mcg/dL (L), and a ferritin of 333 ng/mL (H). Which of the following treatments are indicated in this patient?

a. Oral iron therapy
b. Parenteral iron therapy
c. Erythropoietin therapy
d. Transfusion
e. Better diabetic control

109. You are performing a presurgical clearance evaluation on a 44-year-old otherwise healthy African American male who is undergoing a laproscopic cholecystectomy. His complete blood count (CBC) is shown below:

Hemoglobin: 10.6 g/dL
Mean corpuscular volume: 54 fL (L)
RBC: 6.3 M/uL (H)
Red cell distribution width (RDW): 14.1 (NL)

What should you do prior to surgery?

a. Oral iron replacement for 4 weeks, then recheck before surgery
b. Parenteral iron replacement for 4 weeks, then recheck before surgery
c. Transfusion
d. Hemoglobin electorphoresis
e. Erythropoietin

110. You are evaluating a 26-year-old woman with fatigue. She also complains of lightheadedness, some minor weight loss, and paresthesias in her hands and feet. On examination, her vital signs are normal, but you note pallor and glossitis. Laboratory evaluation reveals a hemoglobin of 9.8 g/dL (L) and a mean corpuscular volume of 102 (H). Which of the following would be most likely to treat her condition?

a. A diet rich in green leafy vegetables
b. A diet rich in iron
c. Vitamin B-12 supplementation
d. Folic acid supplementation
e. Iron supplementation

111. A 68-year-old man complains of fatigue. He has a history of hypertension, well-controlled with hydrochlorothiazide. He's recently lost 30 lb on a high protein, low carbohydrate diet. He drinks 2–3 beers daily, and smokes half pack of cigarettes daily. Laboratory evaluation reveals a macrocytic anemia and vitamin B-12 deficiency. What is the most likely cause?

a. Side effects of hydrochlorothiazide
b. High protein diet
c. Low carbohydrate diet
d. Alcohol intake
e. Inadequate vitamin B-12 absorption

112. A 3-year-old African American male is brought in by his parents with inconsolable crying. He reports extreme pain in his hands and upper extremities. Laboratory evaluation reveals a hemoglobin of 8.2 mg/dL. His peripheral blood smear is as follows:

(Reproduced, with permission, from McPhee S, Papadakis M, and Tierney L. Current Medical Diagnosis and Treatment 2007, 46th ed. New York: McGraw-Hill, 2007.)

Which of the following measures would be most likely to reduce these events in the future?

a. Chronic use of analgesics
b. Adequate hydration
c. Immunization against streptococcal pneumonia
d. Monthly transfusions
e. Daily penicillin prophylaxis until the age of 5

113. You are seeing a 25-year-old male with a rash. It began as pink spots on his extremities, but the lesions have begun to coalesce and become purple in color. He recently returned from a hiking trip in the western mountains. Of the following, which is the most likely cause?

a. Lyme disease
b. Rocky Mountain spotted fever
c. Tularemia
d. Brown recluse spider bite
e. Black widow spider bite

114. You are caring for a person who recently visited New England, and returns with symptoms suggestive of a bite. Which of the following arachnid-bourne illnesses is most likely to occur in the Northeastern United States?

a. Lyme disease
b. Rocky Mountain spotted fever
c. Tularemia
d. Brown recluse spider bite
e. Chigger bites

115. You are seeing a patient who is complaining of an itching scalp. There are erythematous papules on her scalp, and you note small black bulbs at the bases of several hair follicles. Which is the most likely cause of this itch?

a. Flea infestation
b. Bedbugs
c. Head lice
d. Scabies
e. Chigger bites

116. A 26-year-old elementary school teacher presents to you with an itchy rash. You note pruritic erythematous papules in between her fingers, on her wrists, and around her waist at the belt line. Which of the following is the most likely cause?

a. Chigger bites
b. Bedbugs
c. Flea infestation
d. Scabies
e. Body lice

117. While you are working in the emergency room, a 17-year-old patient presents with a cat bite. He was helping a neighbor get his cat out of a tree 3 hours ago, and was bitten on the forearm. On examination, you note erythema, a puncture wound with a jagged laceration, mild purulent discharge, but no tendon involvement. You irrigate the wound thoroughly. What additional therapy is indicated?

a. Hospitalization
b. Human rabies immune globulin
c. Amoxicillin/clavulanic acid
d. Clindamycin
e. Primary closure with subcutaneous sutures

118. A 20-year-old man presents to you 30 minutes after being stung by a bee on his right thigh. He was stung by a bee twice last year. The first sting caused a 3 cm by 3 cm area of erythema, induration and pain around the sting site. The second sting caused a similar 5 cm by 7 cm area. When you examine him, he has an expanding 2 cm by 2 cm area of erythema, induration and pain around the sting site on his thigh. He reports pruritis, fatigue and some nausea, but denies dyspnea. Which of the following is true?

a. This is a typical local reaction, and should spontaneously resolve within hours
b. This is a large local reaction, and the patient has minimal risk for the development of anaphylaxis upon subsequent exposure
c. This is a large local reaction, and the patient is at significant risk for the development of anaphylaxis upon subsequent exposure
d. This is considered a toxic systemic reaction, and increases his risk for anaphylaxis if he is exposed in the future
e. This is considered a mild anaphylactic reaction

119. A 15-year-old male comes to your office complaining of bilateral breast enlargement. He is otherwise healthy and on no medications. On examination, there is mildly tender palpable breast tissue bilaterally. The rest of his physical examination, including his testicular examination is normal. Which of the following is true?

a. No further workup is necessary
b. Serum liver studies are needed to elucidate the cause
c. Thyroid function assessment is needed to elucidate the cause
d. Serum estradiol, testosterone, and leutinizing hormone levels are needed to elucidate the cause
e. His serum chorionic gonadotropin level is likely to be elevated

120. A 22-year-old woman is seeing her physician with complaints of breast pain. It is associated with her menstrual cycle and is described as a bilateral "heaviness" that radiates to the axillae and arms. Examination reveals groups of small breast nodules in the upper outer quadrants of each breast. They are freely mobile and slightly tender. Which of the following statements is most correct?

a. The patient has bilateral fibroadenomas, and reassurance is all that is necessary
b. The patient has bilateral fibroadenomas, and a mammogram is necessary for further evaluation
c. The patient has bilateral fibrocystic changes, and reassurance is all that is necessary
d. The patient has bilateral fibrocystic changes, and a mammogram is necessary for further evaluation
e. The patient has bilateral mastitis, and antibiotic therapy is needed

121. A 35-year-old woman presents to you concerned about a breast mass. Examination reveals no skin changes, diffusely nodular breasts bilaterally with a more dominant, firm, nontender fixed nodule on the left side. The nodule is approximately 7 mm in size, in the upper outer quadrant of the left breast. Her mammogram is negative. Which of the following statements is true?

a. The patient should be reassured and resume routine care
b. The mass should be closely followed with repeat mammogram in 3–6 months
c. The patient should undergo testing for breast cancer genetic mutations, and base further workup on the results
d. The patient should be referred for an ultrasound and possible biopsy
e. If clear amber fluid is aspirated from the mass, it is likely benign, and no further workup is necessary

122. A 28-year-old woman comes to see you for a tender and erythematous area on her breast. She is nursing her 6-week-old son. You diagnose mastitis. Which of the following is true regarding this condition?

a. Restricting caffeine and methylxanthines may be efficacious
b. Evening primrose oil has been shown to help with symptoms
c. Applying ice several times a day will help relieve symptoms
d. The patient should discontinue nursing
e. Antibiotic therapy is indicated

123. You are seeing a 36-year-old woman with a complaint of nipple discharge. Which of the following characteristics of the discharge is most suspicious for breast cancer?

a. Spontaneous discharge
b. Green discharge
c. Bilateral discharge
d. Discharge associated with menses
e. Bloody discharge

124. On screening physical examination of a 36-year-old woman, you find a single left breast mass. It is 1 cm in size, firm, smooth, and apparently fixed to the underlying tissue. You perform a mammogram which is characterized as BI-RADS 3. What does this indicate?

a. The physician should continue routine screening at the usual intervals
b. The physician should perform additional tests (spot compression mammogram, ultrasound) to evaluate the mass as soon as possible
c. The physician should perform diagnostic mammogram of the left breast in 6 months
d. Tissue diagnosis is needed
e. The mass is almost certainly cancerous

125. You are evaluating a 21-year-old woman with an erythematous, tender, and edematous hand. She reports that while playing with her cat 3 days ago, he bit her and punctured the skin. The area around the bite is inflamed, and there is a purulent discharge from the puncture site. What is the most likely infecting organism?

a. *Clostridium perfringens*
b. *Staphylococcus aureus*
c. *Streptococcus pyogenes*
d. *Pasteurella multocida*
e. *Haemophilus influenzae*

126. You are evaluating a 22-year-old male patient who has recently developed a red rash. He just returned from a 4-day skiing trip, where he and his friends used the hot tub at the ski lodge daily. On examination, you note red dome-shaped pustules involving the hair follicles. What is the likely cause of his rash?

a. Streptococcal infection of the hair follicles
b. Staphylococcal infection of the hair follicles
c. Pseudomonal infection of the hair follicles
d. Tinea infection of the hair follicles
e. Candidal infection of the hair follicles

127. You are seeing a 7-month-old boy whose mother is concerned about lesions under his nose and on his upper lip. He has had a runny nose for the last 7 days, but his mother thought that was just a cold. Over the last 2 days, he has developed well-demarcated areas of erythema that seem to have ruptured. The crusts over the lesions are golden yellow. What is the likely cause of this child's lesions?

a. Rhinoviral superficial skin infection
b. Streptococcal superficial skin infection
c. Pseudomonal superficial skin infection
d. *Haemophilus* superficial skin infection
e. Pneumococcal superficial skin infection

128. You are seeing a 15-year-old Caucasian male for acne treatment. Examination of his face reveals multiple closed and open comedones without surrounding erythema or pustules. There is no evidence of scarring. Of the following, what treatment is likely to be most effective for him?

a. Topical antibiotic therapy
b. Oral antibiotic therapy
c. Topical retinoids
d. Prescription strength benzoyl peroxide
e. Oral isotretinoin (Accutane)

129. You are seeing a 14-year-old high school wrestler for a skin condition. About a week ago, he noted a patch of erythematous skin on his right thigh. The patch has enlarged since he first noted it, and the central part of the lesion seems to be crusting and flaking. He reports that it is mildly pruritic. You scrape the lesion and evaluate the shavings under the microscope using potassium hydroxide. You visualize the following:

(Reproduced, with permission, from Wolff K, Johnson RA, Suurmond D. Fitzpatrick's Color Atlas and Synopsis of Clinical Dermatology, 5th ed. New York: McGraw-Hill, 2005: 689.)

What is the most likely diagnosis?

a. Tinea corpris
b. Tinea cruris
c. Pityriasis rosea
d. Numular eczema
e. Impetigo

130. You are evaluating a 40-year-old male patient in the office who is complaining of chest pain. His father had a myocardial infarction at age 42, and the patient is quite concerned. Which characteristic, if included in the history, decreases the likelihood that his chest pain is cardiac in origin?

a. The pain is worse with inspiration
b. The pain radiates to his right arm
c. The pain radiates to his left arm
d. The pain is associated with nausea
e. The pain is associated with sweatiness

131. You are evaluating a 26-year-old female smoker who developed chest pain several hours ago. Her past history is unremarkable, and she takes no medications regularly. She reports the abrupt onset of nonexertional chest pain, associated with shortness of breath and cough. It seems to be worse when she is lying down. It was not brought on by trauma. Which of the following is the most likely origin of her pain?

a. Costochondritis
b. Asthma
c. Pulmonary embolus (PE)
d. Myocardial ischemia
e. Bronchitis

132. You are evaluating a 61-year-old man in the office who is complaining of chest pain. Given his history and risk factors, you are concerned about myocardial ischemia. Which of the following features, if present, would most reliably establish cardiac ischemia as a cause?

a. Relief of pain with nitroglycerine administration
b. Relief of pain with a "gastrointestinal (GI) cocktail" (viscous lidocaine and an antacid)
c. Relief of pain with cessation of activity
d. Relief of pain with eating
e. Relief of pain with sitting up and leaning forward

133. You are evaluating a 20-year-old man presenting to your office with the abrupt onset of chest pain. He has an unremarkable past medical history, but his father had his first myocardial infarction in his late 30s. On examination, he is thin and anxious-appearing. Other than tachycardia, his cardiac examination is normal. His lung examination reveals decreased breath sounds on the right, with hyperresonance to percussion. What is the best treatment for his condition?

a. Insertion of a chest tube
b. Antibiotic therapy
c. Bronchodilator therapy
d. Long-term anticoagulation
e. 325 mg of aspirin immediately, and transfer to an emergency room

134. A nurse asks you to emergently see a patient who came to the office in distress without an appointment. He is 22 years old and is presenting with chest pain. He has never experienced this in the past, and is clearly agitated and upset. He reports a history of slightly elevated blood pressure, "heartburn," and says he is recovering from a recent viral upper respiratory infection. He admits to smoking one pack of cigarettes a day, and has used illegal drugs in the past. His blood pressure is 138/90, and physical examination is significant for tachycardia and diaphoresis. Which of his historical features are most suggestive of myocardial ischemia as a cause of his symptoms?

a. History of hypertension
b. History of "heartburn"
c. Recent viral upper respiratory infection
d. Smoking history
e. Drug use

135. A 45-year-old man with no significant past medical history presents to your office complaining of midsternal chest pain for 5 days. The pain is described as "sharp." On examination, the patient has normal breath sounds, but the pain increases with palpation. Which of the following is the most appropriate next step?

a. Obtain a chest x-ray
b. Obtain a CBC and blood cultures
c. Obtain an electrocardiogram (ECG)
d. Treat with NSAIDs
e. Treat with a proton pump inhibitor

136. A 43-year-old woman with a history of well-controlled hypertension and diabetes presents to your office complaining of intermittent chest pain for the last 3 months. The last episode was 1 week ago, after climbing four flights of stairs at work. The pain was relieved with rest. An ECG in your office is shown below:

(Reproduced, with permission, from Ferry D. Basic Electrocardiography in Ten Days, 1st ed. New York: McGraw-Hill, 2001: 35.)

She is currently asymptomatic. Which of the following is the most appropriate next step?

a. Reassure the patient and have her return if symptoms continue
b. Reassure the patient, but increase her medication to ensure tight control of her blood pressure and glucose levels
c. Admit to the hospital for serial enzymes
d. Obtain a treadmill stress ECG
e. Obtain a treadmill stress echocardiogram

137. You are evaluating a 75-year-old woman with diabetes and hyperlipidemia complaining of chest pain. She reports having occasional chest pain with exertion for years, but yesterday she reported syncope with the pain. On examination, she is afebrile with mildly elevated blood pressure. Cardiac auscultation demonstrates a harsh, rasping crescendo-decrescendo systolic murmur heard best at the second intercostal space at the right upper sternal border. Her carotid pulse is small and rises slowly. Which of the following is the most likely diagnosis?

a. PE
b. Aortic dissection
c. Left ventricular hypertrophy
d. Aortic stenosis
e. Mitral valve prolapse

138. You are evaluating a generally healthy 45-year-old man who is complaining of chest pain. His symptoms are typical for angina, and are relieved with rest. He is a nonsmoker, has no family history of heart disease, but has high cholesterol. His physical examination and ECG are normal. What is the most appropriate next step?

a. Exercise ECG testing
b. Exercise echocardiography
c. Pharmacologic myocardial perfusion imaging
d. Cardiac catheterization
e. Electron beam computed tomography

139. One of your patients is undergoing stress testing for episodic chest pain. He is hypertensive and takes hydrochlorothiazide and metoprolol. Which of the following is the most appropriate advice to give this patient prior to undergoing the stress test?

a. Continue all medications as directed
b. Do not take either antihypertensive medication on the day of the test
c. Continue the metoprolol, but do not take hydrochlorozide at least 2 days before the test
d. Continue hydrocholothiazide, but withdraw the metoprolol at least 2 days before the test
e. Continue hydrochlorothiazide, but withdraw the metoprolol at least 6 days before the test

140. You are seeing a 44-year-old nonsmoker for an acute cough. The cough has been present for 4 days. He had a low-grade fever for the first 2 days, but that has resolved. He reports that the cough is worse at night, has become productive of yellow sputum, but there is no hemoptysis or shortness of breath. What is the most likely cause of the cough?

a. Pneumonia
b. Sinusitis with postnasal drip
c. Pertussis
d. Viral upper respiratory infection
e. Tuberculosis

141. A 33-year-old nonsmoking man presents to you for evaluation of his chronic cough. He says the cough has been present for about 8 weeks. Initially, he went to an urgent care where he received antitussives and a bronchodilator. Those did not help, and he returned 1 week later and was given a course of azithromycin. His cough has continued to persist. His symptoms are worse when he lies down for sleep, and are associated with a sore throat and a "sour" taste in the back of his mouth. He has also noticed that when he drinks caffeine or alcohol, the cough seems to worsen. What is the most likely diagnosis?

a. Gastroesophageal reflux
b. Asthma
c. Side effect from a medicaiton
d. Chronic bronchitis
e. Pertussis

142. You are treating a 52-year-old woman with a 40-pack/year history of smoking. She reports a productive cough that has been present for the last 3–4 months, beginning in the fall. She remembers having the same symptoms last year in the fall, and attributed it to a "cold that she just couldn't kick." She does not have fevers, reports mild dyspnea when walking up stairs, and denies hempotysis. What is the most likely diagnosis?

a. Irritation of airways from cigarette smoke
b. Chronic bronchitis
c. Postnasal drainage due to seasonal allergies
d. Lung cancer
e. Asthma

143. Four weeks ago, you treated a 22-year-old woman for acute bronchitis. Although she feels much better, the cough has persisted. She has used bronchodilators, antihistamines, and antitussives. What is the best course of treatment at this time?

a. A 10-day course of amoxicillin
b. A 5-day course of azithromycin
c. Steroid nasal spray
d. NSAIDs
e. An oral steroid taper

144. You are seeing an 18-year-old man who has had a cough for 2 weeks. It started like a typical "cold," but has persisted. Over the last 3 days, the cough has come in "spasms" and he barely has time to catch his breath during the coughing episodes. Nasopharyngeal swab confirms the diagnosis of pertussis. Which of the following treatments is recommended?

a. A 10-day course of amoxicillin
b. A 10-day course of amoxicillin/clavulanate
c. A 10-day course of erythromycin
d. A 5-day course of azithromycin
e. Supportive therapy without antibiotics, but in isolation

145. You are seeing a 6-month-old boy whose mother reports that he has had diarrhea for almost 2 weeks. He has had 4–6 bowel movements a day, with a loose to liquid consistency. His mother stays at home with him and the child is not in daycare. His symptoms began after his young cousins visited for Christmas. What would be the most likely cause of his diarrhea?

a. Rotavirus
b. Norwalk virus
c. Giardiasis
d. *Salmonella*
e. *Enterotoxigenic E. coli*

146. A 25-year-old woman returned from her honeymoon in Mexico yesterday. She spent the last day of her trip with frequent loose bowel movements that have persisted over this 3-day period. She has not had fevers or blood in her stool. Her examination is unremarkable. What is most likely cause of her diarrhea?

a. Rotavirus
b. Norwalk virus
c. Giardiasis
d. *Salmonella*
e. Enterotoxigenic *E. coli*

147. You have diagnosed travelers' diarrhea in a 30-year-old otherwise healthy man who has recently returned from an African safari. Which of the following is the best empiric treatment option?

a. Erythromycin
b. Ciprofloxacin
c. Metronidazole
d. Doxycycline
e. Vancomycin

148. A 28-year-old mother of two young children is seeing you to discuss her chronic diarrhea. She reports that symptoms began in her early 20s. She doesn't have symptoms daily, but does report at least 1 day a week with more frequent bowel movements with a less firm consistency. She reports crampy abdominal pain that is relieved with bowel movements, passage of some mucus with bowel movements, a sensation of incomplete evacuation and abdominal distention. She denies nighttime symptoms, does not note symptoms with certain foods or liquids, has not lost weight, and has never passed blood with her stools. What is the most likely cause of her diarrhea?

a. Giardiasis
b. *Entamoeba histolytica*
c. Irritable bowel syndrome (IBS)
d. Inflammatory bowel disease
e. Lactose intolerance

149. You have diagnosed an otherwise healthy adult with acute viral diarrhea. Which of the following dietary measures should you recommend?

a. The patient should fast until the diarrhea resolves
b. The patient should not eat solids, but should drink an oral rehydrating solution
c. The patient should drink milk
d. The patient should avoid wheat, barley, and rye.
e. The patient should avoid caffeine

150. A 33-year-old woman is seeing you with a chief complaint of "dizziness." Upon further characterization, she describes "unsteadiness" and a feeling that "her balance is off." Based on this description, which of the following terms should be used to characterize her complaint?

a. Vertigo
b. Orthostasis
c. Presyncope
d. Dysequilibrium
e. Lightheadedness

151. A 42-year-old woman is seeing you to follow up with a new complaint of "dizziness." She reports that symptoms first began several months ago. At that time, she reported a subjective hearing loss and a ringing in her left ear only. Symptoms were mild, and her physical examination was normal, so you elected to follow her. Since that time, her symptoms have progressed to include dizziness and some facial numbness. What is her most likely diagnosis?

a. Vestibular neuronitis
b. Benign positional vertigo
c. Acoustic neuroma
d. Meniere's disease
e. Cerebellar tumor

152. In the evaluation of a 55-year-old man complaining of dizziness, you perform the Dix-Hallpike (Nylen-Barany) maneuver several times. You had the patient sit on the edge of the examining table and lie down suddenly with the head hanging 45° backward and turned to either side. With this maneuver, the vertigo was reproduced immediately, and symptoms did not lessen regardless of repetition. The direction of the nystagmus changed with changing the direction that the head is turned, and the symptoms were of mild intensity. Which of the following is the most likely cause of the vertigo?

a. Stroke
b. Vestibular neuronitis
c. Benign positional vertigo
d. Meinere's disease
e. Acoustic neuroma

153. You are caring for a 26-year-old man with vertigo. You have diagnosed him with a peripheral vestibular disorder, and are considering treatment options. Which of the following would be the first-line therapy?

a. NSAIDs
b. Antihistamines
c. Antiemetics
d. Antibiotics
e. Benzodiazepines

154. You are evaluating a patient complaining of "dizziness," but your history and examination cannot distinguish whether his symptoms are suggestive of a central or peripheral cause. Which of the following tests is the best option for clarification?

a. MRI of the brain
b. CT scan of the brain
c. Audiometry
d. Brainstem evoked audiometry
e. Electronystagmography

155. You are evaluating a 56-year-old farmer who is complaining of dyspnea. His history includes being hospitalized for bronchiolitis as a young child leading to childhood asthma, and a history of pneumonia 2 years ago, for which he was also hospitalized. He has a 20-pack year history of smoking. Which of the following increase his risk for having restrictive lung disease as the cause of his dyspnea?

a. A history of childhood bronchiolitis
b. A history of asthma
c. A smoking history
d. A recent history of pneumonia
e. His occupation as a farmer

156. You are seeing a 26-year-old female patient complaining of dyspnea. She reports having an upper respiratory infection 2–3 weeks ago, but that seemed to resolve. Since then, she has noted progressive weakness of the muscles in her legs, and yesterday began feeling short of breath. She is worse today. On examination, she has symmetric proximal leg muscle weakness with markedly depressed deep tendon reflexes. Her lung examination is significant for decreased inspiratory volume without crackles or wheezes. What is her most likely diagnosis?

a. Parkinson's disease
b. Gullain-Barre syndrome
c. Amyotrophic lateral sclerosis
d. Lyme disease
e. Psychogenic weakness and dyspnea

157. You are evaluating a 36-year-old woman with dyspnea. She reports a cough and some pleuritic chest pain. On examination, her temperature is 101°F, and you note egophony in the left lower lobe. What is the likely cause of the dyspnea?

a. Asthma
b. Bronchitis
c. Pneumonia
d. PE
e. Congestive heart failure (CHF)

158. You are evaluating a 71-year-old male patient with the complaint of shortness of breath. It mainly occurs with exertion. He also complains of fatigue, and needing to sleep propped up on two pillows. On physical examination, you note a large apical impulse and jugular venous distension (JVD). He has fine crackles in the bases of both lungs with decreased breath sounds. What would be the most appropriate treatment?

a. Bronchodilators
b. Antibiotics
c. Steroids
d. Anticoagulation
e. Diuretics

159. You are seeing a young child whose mother says she is having trouble breathing. She is 3 years old, and this is her third episode of difficulty breathing. On examination, you note nasal flaring and sternal retractions with accessory muscle use. You auscultate expiratory wheezes bilaterally. Which of the following is the most likely diagnosis?

a. Bronchiolitis
b. Asthma
c. Pneumonia
d. Ventricular septal defect
e. Valvular disease

160. You are seeing a 23-year-old woman with the complaint of shortness of breath. She is otherwise healthy, taking only oral contraceptives regularly. The dyspnea began suddenly, and is associated with pleuritic chest pain. On physical examination, you note tachypnea, tachycardia, and some mild unilateral lower extremity edema. What would the best treatment option be for this patient?

a. Bronchodilators
b. Antibiotics
c. Steroids
d. Anticoagulation
e. Diuretics

161. You are evaluating a 69-year-old woman with a history of asthma and ischemic cardiomyopathy who is complaining of dyspnea. You are not sure if her symptoms are related to asthma or CHF, and you order a b-type natriuretic peptide to help in her evaluation. The level is found to be 76 pg/mL (normal is 0–100 pg/mL). Which of the following is most correct regarding the interpretation of this laboratory value?

a. The probability that her symptoms are related to CHF is near zero
b. The probability that her symptoms are related to CHF is low
c. The probability that her symptoms are related to CHF is moderate
d. The probability that her symptoms are related to CHF is high
e. The probability that her symptoms are related to CHF is indeterminate

162. You are seeing a sedentary, obese 41-year-old woman who presents to you with acute shortness of breath. She has tachycardia, but no other abnormal examination findings. You order a d-dimer and it comes back low. Which of the following is the most appropriate option?

a. Order a spiral CT of the chest
b. Order a ventilation/perfusion (V/Q) scan
c. Order Doppler flow studies of her lower extremities
d. Order a pulmonary angiogram
e. Reassure the patient

163. One of your patients is dying of end stage breast cancer. She is complaining of dyspnea. Which of the following treatment options would be most beneficial?

a. Bronchodilators
b. Steroids
c. Anxiolytics
d. Opioids
e. A pulmonary rehabilitation program

164. A 23-year-old sexually active woman visits a free clinic, reporting a sudden onset of dysuria that began 2 days ago. On further questioning, she also reports urinary frequency, some back pain, and a pink discoloration to her urine. She denies vaginal discharge or irritation, and has been afebrile. The clinic has no microscope or urine dip sticks available. Based on this history, what is her most likely diagnosis?

a. Acute bacterial cystitis
b. Urethritis
c. Pyelonephritis
d. Interstitial cystitis
e. Vulvovaginitis

165. An 18-year-old woman is seeing you for back pain, frequency, and dysuria. She has never had a urinary tract infection (UTI) in the past, and though she recently became sexually active, she denies vaginal discharge or risk for sexually transmitted infection. In this setting, when would a urine culture be necessary?

a. If a urine dipstick were negative
b. If a urine dipstick was positive for leukocyte esterase only
c. If a urine dipstick was positive for leukocyte esterase and blood
d. If a microscopic evaluation of her centrifuged urine revealed more than 5 white blood cells per high powered field
e. If a microscopic evaluation of her centrifuged urine revealed significant bacteriuria

166. You are evaluating a 25-year-old woman who reports frequent UTIs since getting married last year. In the last 12 months, she has had 5 documented infections that have responded well to antibiotic therapy. She has tried voiding after intercourse, she discontinued her use of a diaphragm, and tried acidification of her urine using oral ascorbic acid, but none of those measures decreased the incidence of infections. At this point, which of the following would be an acceptable prophylactic measure?

a. An antibiotic prescription for the usual 3-day regimen with refills, to be used when symptoms occur
b. Single dose antibiotic therapy once daily at bedtime for 12 months
c. Single dose antibiotic therapy once daily at bedtime for 2 years
d. Single dose antibiotic therapy after sexual intercourse
e. Antibiotics for 3 days after sexual intercourse

167. A 36-year-old woman comes to your office complaining of recurrent dysuria. This is her fourth episode in the past 10 months. Initially, her symptoms were "classic" for a UTI. She was treated without obtaining urine dipstick or microscopic evaluation. For the second episode, her urinalysis was positive for blood only. Her culture was negative, as was evaluation for nephrolithiasis. The third episode was similar, also with a negative culture. All episodes have resolved with a standard course of antibiotic therapy. What should you do at this time?

a. Evaluate for somatization disorder
b. Order cystoscopy
c. Treat for chronic vaginitis
d. Use a 14-day regimen of antibiotics
e. Use daily single dose antibiotic therapy for prophylaxis

168. A screening urinalysis in a female patient reveals asymptomatic bacteriuria. In which of the following patients would treatment be indicated?

a. A sexually active teenager
b. A pregnant 26-year-old
c. A 45-year-old with uncontrolled hypertension
d. A menopausal woman
e. An otherwise healthy 80-year-old woman

169. You are seeing a 34-year-old man with urinary symptoms. He reports frequency, urgency, and moderate back pain. He is febrile and acutely ill. He has no penile discharge. His urinalysis shows marked pyuria. He has never had an episode like this before, and has no known urinary tract abnormalities. What is the most likely diagnosis?

a. Gonococcal urethritis
b. Nongonococcal urethritis
c. Acute bacterial cystitis
d. Pyelonephritis
e. Acute prostatitis

170. You are seeing a child with a chief complaint of ear pain. Which of the following would be considered a risk factor for acute otitis media?

a. Age between 6 months and 7 years
b. Caucasian race
c. History of a heart murmur
d. Parents with seasonal allergies
e. Child cared for by a babysitter at home while the parents are at work

171. A 26-year-old man presents to his physician with a complaint of left ear pain and associated hearing loss on that side. Which of the following is *least* likely to be a cause?

a. Acute otitis media
b. Eustacean tube dysfunction
c. Barotrauma
d. Severe otitis externa
e. Temporomandibular joint syndrome

172. You are seeing a 25-year-old patient complaining of a left sided earache. She describes the pain as deep, and worse with eating. Her ear examination is normal, but she has tenderness and crepitus during palpation of the left temporomandibular joint. Which of the following would be the most appropriate next step?

a. Antibiotic therapy
b. Treatment with NSAIDs
c. Dental referral
d. MRI of the temporomandibular joint
e. Obtaining an erythrocyte sedimentation rate

173. The mother of a 9-month-old infant brings him in for irritability. The child has been fussy and has not been sleeping well for 2 days. His highest temperature has been 100°F, and he has had a clear runny nose and a cough. On examination, the child is crying and irritable. Which physical examination finding, by itself, is *least* likely to be helpful in diagnosing acute otitis media?

a. An opaque tympanic membrane
b. A bulging tympanic membrane
c. Impaired tympanic membrane mobility
d. An erythematous tympanic membrane
e. Purulent discharge in the ear canal

174. You are seeing a 4-year-old male 2 weeks after being diagnosed with left acute otitis media. He completed his therapy, is afebrile, acting well, and apparently back to normal. On examination, he has a persistent effusion in the left ear. There is no erythema, purulence or hearing loss. Of the following, which is the most appropriate next step?

a. Reassurance and reevaluation in 2–4 weeks
b. A 10-day course of a second-line antibiotic
c. Regular use of a decongestant and reevaluation in 2 weeks
d. Regular use of an antihistamine and reevaluation in 2 weeks
e. Referral to an otolaryngologist

175. You are seeing a 2-year-old with recurrent ear infections. His three older siblings also had frequent ear infections. He is in daycare 4 days a week, and he has not had immunizations since 4 months of age. He continues to use a pacifier. Based on his history, which of the following is his most significant risk factor for otitis media?

a. Family history of otitis media
b. Daycare
c. The number of siblings in the household
d. Inadequate vaccination
e. Pacifier use

176. You are seeing a 35-year-old woman who complains of ear pain. She has a history of bruxism and dental malocclusion, and has had no response to nonsteroidal anti-inflammatory treatment. What would be the next step in treating for her problem?

a. Penicillin
b. Azithromycin
c. Corticosteroids
d. Referral for a bite guard
e. Physical therapy

177. You are seeing a 6-year-old patient whose mother brought him in for ear pain and fever. On examination, he is febrile, and his right tympanic membrane is shown below:

(Reproduced, with permission, from Knoop K, Stack L, Storrow A. Atlas of Emergency Medicine, 2nd ed. New York: McGraw-Hill, 2002: 118.)

Which of the following would be the best initial treatment?

a. A weight adjusted dose of Tylenol
b. A weight adjusted course of amoxicillin
c. A weight adjusted one-time dose of azithromycin
d. A weight adjusted 3-day course of azithromycin
e. A weight adjusted 5-day course of azithromycin

178. You are talking with a mother of three young children, ages 2 months, 3 years, and 5 years. The 3- and 5-year-olds have a history of recurrent acute otitis media, and both of them have required tympanostomy tubes. She asks about pneumococcal vaccination to help prevent ear infections in her infant. Which of the following is true regarding the effect of vaccination on the cases of acute otitis media?

a. The vaccination is associated with about a 10% reduction in cases of recurrent acute otitis media
b. The vaccination is associated with about a 20% reduction in cases of recurrent acute otitis media

c. The vaccination is associated with about a 30% reduction in cases of recurrent acute otitis media

d. The vaccination is associated with about a 50% reduction in cases of recurrent acute otitis media

e. The vaccination is associated with about a 80% reduction in cases of recurrent acute otitis media

179. You are seeing an 18-year-old college athlete complaining of ear pain. His pain has been present for 4 days, and seems to be worsening. He has no fever or symptoms of upper respiratory infection. On examination, his ear canal is tender, erythematous, and swollen. His tympanic membrane is obscured by discharge and debris. What is the treatment of choice for this patient?

a. Flushing of the ear canal with hydrogen peroxide
b. Topical antibiotics
c. Systemic antibiotics
d. Topical hydrocortisone
e. Oral steroids

180. You are seeing a 45-year-old diabetic woman who reports bilateral lower extremity peripheral edema. In addition to diabetes, she has hypertension and depression. Which of the following medications is the likely cause of her edema?

a. Fluoxetine
b. Metformin
c. Rosiglitazone
d. Lisinopril
e. Hydrochlorothiazide

181. You are seeing a 23-year-old woman complaining of swelling of the lower legs. On examination, you note lower leg edema that spares the feet. What is the likely cause?

a. Lymphedema
b. Lipedema
c. Hepatocellular disease
d. Venous insufficiency
e. Varicose veins

182. You are evaluating a 47-year-old woman complaining of bilateral lower extremity edema. She denies dyspnea, and on examination has no rales, JVD, or ascites. Her cardiac examination is normal. What would be the next step in the evaluation of her edema?

a. Echocardiogram
b. Thyroid stimulating hormone
c. Liver function studies
d. A lower extremity Doppler
e. A urinalysis

183. You are evaluating a 40-year-old woman with a new onset of bilateral lower extremity edema. She denies dyspnea, and on examination has no rales or JVD. On evaluation, she has an abdominal fluid wave. Which of the following would be the next step in the evaluation of her edema?

a. Echocardiogram
b. Thyroid stimulating hormone
c. Liver function tests
d. A lower extremity Doppler
e. A urinalysis

184. You are evaluating a 33-year-old obese man who noted unilateral lower extremity edema. He denies dyspnea or recent trauma. On evaluation, you note pitting edema on the right without signs of trauma, erythema, or inflammation. Which of the following would be the most appropriate next step in the evaluation of his edema?

a. Echocardiogram
b. Thyroid stimulating hormone
c. Liver function studies
d. A lower extremity Doppler
e. A urinalysis

185. You are evaluating a 63-year-old diabetic man who noted unilateral lower extremity edema. He denies dyspnea or recent trauma. On evaluation, you note pitting edema on the right with well-demarcated erythema from the ankle to the midthigh. Which of the following is the most likely diagnosis?

a. Varicose veins
b. Chronic CHF
c. Venous insufficiency
d. Deep venous thrombosis (DVT)
e. Cellulitis

186. You are evaluating a 55-year-old man with hypertension and hyper-lipidemia who complains of unilateral lower extremity edema. It has been present on and off for almost a year. He denies dyspnea or recent trauma, and has no evidence of inflammation. Which of the following would the best treatment option for his condition?

a. Diuresis
b. Anticoagulation
c. Elastic stockings
d. Sodium restriction
e. An angiotensin converting enzyme (ACE) inhibitor

187. You are evaluating a 5-year-old girl brought in by her parents to dis-cuss eneuresis. She was toilet trained in the daytime at the age of 3 years, and was dry at night at about 3½ years of age. Four months ago, her par-ents had another child, and the 5-year-old began to wet the bed at night. She has no medical condition that would account for the change. What term correctly describes this condition?

a. Primary nocturnal enuresis
b. Primary diurnal enuresis
c. Secondary nocturnal enuresis
d. Secondary diurnal enuresis
e. Primary intentional enuresis

188. You are seeing a 6-year-old girl whose parents brought her in to have her bedwetting evaluated. She has been toilet trained during the day since the age of 4, but still wets the bed at night. Her father wet the bed until the age of 8 years. Her physical examination reveals no abnormalities, and her urinalysis is normal. Which of the following statements is true regarding this situation?

a. Up to 20% of 6-year-olds are enuretic
b. Her father's history is inconsequential in this situation
c. It is unusual for young girls to have a problem with enuresis
d. The problem is likely due to her being a deeper sleeper than other children
e. There is likely an organic cause to her problem

189. You are counseling a parent whose 7-year-old son wets the bed at night. Which intervention has proven to be the most effective for this condition?

a. Frequent night-time wakening to encourage voiding
b. Use of an alarm that wakes the child when he wets at night
c. Use of desmopressin (synthetic DDAVP)
d. Use of tricyclic antidepressant medications (e.g., imipramine)
e. Use of an anticholinergic antispasmodic (e.g., oxybutynin)

190. You are evaluating a 6-year-old boy. His mother has brought him in because he wets the bed. He has never been dry at night, and his parents are starting to get concerned. You obtain a thorough voiding history, and find the child to be completely normal on physical examination. He is otherwise developmentally normal. His urinalysis is also normal. What is the next step in the workup of this patient?

a. Observation
b. X-rays of the lumbar and sacral spine
c. Renal ultrasound
d. Voiding cystourethrogram (VCUG)
e. Both renal ultrasound and voiding cystourethrogram

191. One of the children in your practice is troubled by nocturnal enuresis. He is 7 years old, and has avoided overnight activities with friends. Which of the following is the best initial treatment measure?

a. Treatment of constipation
b. Motivational therapy with consequences for not maintaining a dry bed
c. Desmopressin acetate (DDAVP)
d. Imipramine (Tofranil)
e. Tolterodine (Detrol)

192. You are discussing enuresis therapy with the mother of an 8-year-old girl that you care for. She is not interested in pharmacologic therapies, but would like to discuss using a moisture-sensitive alarm. Which of the following is true regarding the use of these alarms for nocturnal enuresis?

a. The goal of this alarm is to wake the child just after the initiation of urination
b. The success rate is greater for boys than for girls
c. The success rate is less than 50%
d. If the process will be successful, it only takes 3–4 weeks on average
e. The alarms are easier for families because the child takes responsibility for the treatment

193. You are seeing a 13-month-old Caucasian male. His growth chart is shown. His past medical history and physical examination are otherwise unremarkable, and he is meeting his developmental milestones. Which of the following is most likely to reveal the cause of his growth pattern?

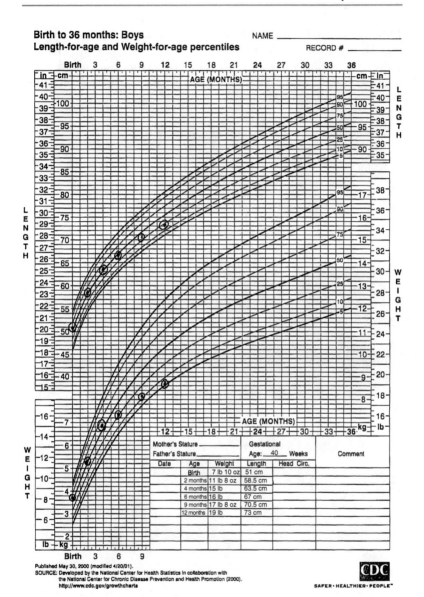

Birth to 36 months: Boys
Length-for-age and Weight-for-age percentiles

NAME _____

RECORD # _____

	Date	Age	Weight	Length	Head Circ.
	Birth		7 lb 10 oz	51 cm	
		2 months	11 lb 8 oz	58.5 cm	
		4 months	15 lb	63.5 cm	
		6 months	16 lb	67 cm	
		9 months	17 lb 8 oz	70.5 cm	
		12 months	19 lb	73 cm	

Mother's Stature _____
Father's Stature _____
Gestational Age: __40__ Weeks
Comment

Published May 30, 2000 (modified 4/20/01).
SOURCE: Developed by the National Center for Health Statistics in collaboration with
the National Center for Chronic Disease Prevention and Health Promotion (2000).
http://www.cdc.gov/growthcharts

CDC
SAFER · HEALTHIER · PEOPLE™

a. A thorough dietary history
b. Serum albumin levels
c. Serum prealbumin levels
d. Assessment of the thyroid stimulating hormone
e. Serum IgA levels

194. You are evaluating a 9-month-old Caucasian girl for poor weight gain. She has gone from the 75th percentile to the 10th percentile in height and weight. She has had recurrent respiratory infections and diarrhea, but cultures obtained have been negative. Which of the following will be the most useful test in this setting?

a. A Mantoux test for tuberculosis
b. Assessment for human immunodeficiency virus
c. Stool for ova and parasites
d. A sweat chloride test
e. Renal function tests

195. You are seeing a 15-month-old for a well-child check. His parents have no concerns and his developmental history is normal. His growth chart is shown.

Which of the following is the most likely?

a. Familial short stature
b. Failure to thrive
c. Hypothyroidism
d. A normal breast-fed infant
e. Constitutional growth delay

Birth to 36 months: Boys
Length-for-age and Weight-for-age percentiles

NAME _ _____

RECORD # _____

Date	Age	Weight	Length	Head Circ.	Comment
	Birth	8 lb 8 oz	20.5 in		
	2 months	12 lb 4 oz	23 in		
	4 months	14 lb 9 oz	25 in		
	6 months	17 lb	26.5 in		
	9 months	19 lb 8 oz	27.5 in		
	12 months	21 lb 6 oz	29 in		
	15 months	22 lb 8 oz	30 in		

Mother's Stature _____
Father's Stature _____
Gestational Age: _____ Weeks

Published May 30, 2000 (modified 4/20/01).
SOURCE: Developed by the National Center for Health Statistics in collaboration with
the National Center for Chronic Disease Prevention and Health Promotion (2000).
http://www.cdc.gov/growthcharts

SAFER · HEALTHIER · PEOPLE™

196. You have been following a 12-month-old infant. At 9 months, his height was at the 25th percentile while his weight was at the 5th percentile. At 12 months, his weight and height are unchanged. His physical examination shows:

Blood pressure: 62/32 (low)
Heart rate: 72 beats per minute
Respiratory rate: 16 per minute
Temperature: 98.8°F

Which is the best therapeutic option for this child?
a. Nutritional instruction to take two times the normal caloric intake
b. Iron supplementation with increased calorie intake
c. Zinc with increased caloric intake
d. Referral to social services for neglect
e. Hospital admission

197. A 19-year-old presented to your office with a 3-day history of fatigue, sore throat, and low-grade fevers. On examination, his temperature was 100.3°F, and you noted an exudative pharyngitis with cervical adenopathy. You sent a throat culture and started him on amoxicillin prophylactically. Two days later, he presents for follow up with continued symptoms and a diffuse, symmetrical erythematous maculopapular rash. What is the most likely cause of his symptoms?
a. Scarlet fever
b. Allergic reaction to amoxicillin
c. Viral exanthem
d. Mononucleosis
e. Measles

198. A 48-year-old man presents with a history of "feeling tired" for about 6 months. His previous doctor told him he probably had chronic fatigue syndrome, and he is presenting to you for a second opinion. He reports that his sleep is not refreshing. He has postexertional fatigue, weight loss, and also reports impaired concentration and headaches. Which of those symptoms is less likely to be associated with chronic fatigue syndrome?
a. Unrefreshing sleep
b. Postexertional fatigue
c. Weight loss
d. Impaired concentration
e. Headaches

199. A 23-year-old woman presents to your office to discuss fatigue. She describes a "lack of energy" and "tiredness," denying weakness or hypersomnolence. What is the next step in the workup?

a. Screen for depression
b. Screen for sleep apnea
c. Screen for anemia
d. Screen for hypothyroidism
e. Screen for pregnancy

200. You are discussing fatigue with one of your 53-year-old patients. She reports that her symptoms have occurred for the past 6 months, and have been getting progressively worse. She reports increased stress and working longer hours at work, and she is drinking a glass of red wine each evening after work to relax. Which component of her history points to a physical cause of her fatigue?

a. Symptoms for 6 months
b. Progressively worsening
c. Associated with increased stress
d. Occurring when working longer hours
e. Alcohol overuse

201. You are evaluating a 55-year-old African American man for fatigue. His history and physical are unremarkable, and your diagnosis is uncertain. What should be included in your initial workup?

a. Chest x-ray
b. ECG
c. HIV test
d. Prostate cancer screen
e. Drug screen

202. A mother brings her son in to see you. He is almost 2 years old, and had a significant amount of painless bleeding from his rectum last evening. He is currently hemodynamically stable, and in no distress when you see him. What is the most likely diagnosis?

a. Juvenile polyposis
b. Colitis
c. Anal fissure
d. Intussusception
e. Meckel's diverticulum

203. A 36-year-old man reports a 1-day history of hematemesis. He is complaining of some mild abdominal pain, but otherwise feels well. He denies alcohol use. On examination, he is tender in the epigastric region without peritoneal signs. His fecal occult blood test is positive, but his stool is not grossly bloody. What is the next step in his workup?

a. Gastric lavage
b. Barium study
c. Endoscopy
d. Red cell scan
e. Angiography

204. You are evaluating a 44-year-old man with painless, large volume intestinal hemorrhage. You suspect a Meckel's diverticulum as the possible cause. What is the best test to confirm this diagnosis?

a. An esophagogastroduodenoscopy
b. A sigmoidoscopy
c. A colonoscopy
d. A technetium-99m pertechnetate scintigraphic study
e. A laparotomy

205. A 56-year-old man is found to have asymptomatic diverticulosis on screening colonoscopy. He is concerned about his risk for GI bleeding from the diverticula. Which of the following statements is most accurate regarding his concern?

a. Severe diverticular bleeding is relatively common, occurring in up to 50% of patients with diverticulosis
b. Diverticular bleeding is usually triggered by the ingestion of nuts, berries, seeds, popcorn, or other relatively indigestible material
c. Diverticular bleeding resolves spontaneously in the vast majority of cases
d. In patients with diverticular bleeding undergoing colonoscopy, blood emanating from a diverticulum is usually seen
e. If colonoscopy fails to localize the source of active bleeding, a subtotal colectomy is needed to ensure no future bleeding

206. You are evaluating a 33-year-old man with rectal pain and bleeding. He reports that he initially felt a mass near his rectum several days ago. It was associated with some bright red blood on the toilet paper when he wiped after a bowel movement. The area became acutely painful over the last 24 hours. On examination, you note an exquisitely tender, purple nodule distal to the dentate line. What is the office-based treatment of choice for his condition?

a. Hydrocortisone suppositories
b. Rubber band ligation
c. Sclerotherapy
d. Incision and drainage
e. Excision

207. You are evaluating a patient in the office with hematochezia. He has had chronic constipation, and reports bright red blood from his rectum associated with extremely painful bowel movements. After defecation, he complains of a dull ache and a feeling of "spasm" in the anal canal. The pain resolves within a few hours. On external examination, no abnormalities are noted. What is his most likely diagnosis?

a. Anal fissure
b. Thrombosed external hemorrhoid
c. Internal hemorrhoid
d. Thrombosed internal hemorrhoid
e. Peri-anal abscess

208. A 23-year-old woman presents to your office complaining of headaches. Which of the following characteristics is more likely to be associated with migraine headaches than other types of headaches?

a. Unilateral symptoms
b. Severe in intensity
c. Nausea
d. Rhinorrhea
e. Sweating

209. You are evaluating a patient with a headache. Of the following, which is the most important in characterizing the type of headache the patient is experiencing?

a. History
b. Physical examination
c. Blood work
d. Imaging
e. Consultation with neurology

210. You are talking with a 24-year-old woman complaining of a headache. She reports that before she has the headache, she experiences visual symptoms associated with slight nausea. When the headache occurs later, it is throbbing, pulsating, and unilateral. During the headache, she experiences light sensitivity. Sleep improves the symptoms. Her symptoms are disrupting her daily life, and you decide to try prophylactic therapy. Which of the following is the most studied prophylactic agent to use?

a. Beta-blockers
b. Calcium channel blockers
c. Selective serotonin reuptake inhibitors
d. Anticonvulsants
e. Ergotamines

211. One of your patients has been on beta-blocker therapy for migraine prophylaxis. Her symptoms are not optimally controlled, and she is interested in other therapies. What agent, when added to the beta-blocker, has a synergistic effect in the prophylaxis of migraines?

a. Calcium channel blockers
b. Tricyclic antidepressants
c. Selective serotonin reuptake inihibitors
d. Anticonvulsants
e. Ergotamines

212. You are caring for a 33-year-old migraine sufferer. He is currently complaining of an acute migraine attack, and is interested in abortive therapy. Which of the following options is *least* likely to be effective?

a. Acetaminophen
b. NSAIDs
c. 5-HT agonists
d. Ergotamines
e. Narcotics

213. You are discussing migraine management with a 30-year-old woman. She wants to use prophylactic medications, but had debilitating fatigue and symptoms of depression on beta-blockers. Which of the following medications is an acceptable alternative?

a. Nifedipine
b. Verapamil
c. Diltiazem
d. Amlodipine
e. Nicardipine

214. A 41-year-old man comes to the office to discuss his headache symptoms. He first began having symptoms a couple of years ago. He describes the headaches dramatically—"like an ice pick is going through my eye!"—and describes it as the worst pain in his life. The headaches begin suddenly, are unilateral, last up to 2 hours, and are associated with runny nose and watery eye. He gets several attacks over a couple of months, but is symptom free for months in-between flare ups. What is the best approach for long term management of the attacks?

a. Fluoxetine, 20–60 mg daily
b. Prednisone, 10 mg daily
c. Indomethacin, 120 mg daily
d. Nifedipine, 40–120 mg daily during the symptomatic period
e. Ergotamine, 1–2 mg daily during the symptomatic period

215. A 40-year-old man transfers to your office from out of state after moving to your community. He suffers from cluster headaches, and would like a medication to manage the acutely painful episodes. Which of the following would be best for treatment of the acute episodes?

a. Indomethacin, 120 mg by mouth
b. Oxycodone, 5–10 mg by mouth
c. Sumatriptan, 50–100 mg by mouth
d. Ergotamine, 1–2 mg by mouth
e. 4% lidocaine, 1 mL administered into the nostril

216. You are talking with a 33-year-old woman who is complaining of headaches. She has had these headaches for 5 months, and they are increasing in frequency. She reports that the headaches may last anywhere from an hour to several days. They are now occurring about 5–10 times a month, without relationship to her menstrual cycle. She describes the headache as bilateral, and the pain is described as a pressure around her forehead. She denies nausea, is not sensitive to sound, but is sensitive to light during an attack. On examination, she has no obvious neurological deficit. What is the best approach to take at this point?

a. Prescribe narcotic analgesics and follow up if no improvement
b. Prescribe NSAIDs and follow up if no improvement
c. Order blood work to rule out secondary cause
d. Order a CT of the brain
e. Order an MRI of the brain

217. You are evaluating a 48-year-old woman with headaches. She reports a long history of occasional sinus headaches, usually responding to over-the-counter treatment. Over the last several months, the headaches are occurring more frequently, and are actually more painful than they have been in the past. Over-the-counter medications, effective in the past, no longer work. What is the most appropriate next step?

a. Use antibiotics to treat sinusitis and follow up if no improvement
b. Use prescription antihistamines and follow up if no improvement
c. Use prescription decongestants and follow up if no improvement
d. Use NSAIDs and follow up if no improvement
e. Obtain radiological imaging of the brain

218. You are taking care of a 36-year-old woman with mild hypertension, arthritis, and depression. She also has been taking daily oral penicillin for a streptococcal throat infection. She notes the acute onset of hematuria, and comes to your office for evaluation. Which of the following medications is most likely to cause this symptom?

a. Ibuprofen
b. Penicillin
c. Fluoxetine
d. Oral contraceptives
e. Hydrochlorothiazide

219. A 16-year-old sexually active woman comes to your office complaining of blood in her urine. She reports suprapubic pain, dysuria, and frequency. What is the likely diagnosis?

a. Cystitis
b. Pyelonephritis
c. Nephrolithiasis
d. Bladder cancer
e. A sexually transmitted infection

220. You are evaluating a 56-year-old generally healthy man who is seeing you after finding blood in his urine. He denies pain, dysuria, frequency, or urgency. He is a smoker, and has worked for years in the printing industry. What is the most likely cause of his hematuria?

a. Acute prostatitis
b. Chronic prostatitis
c. A UTI
d. Urinary stones
e. Bladder carcinoma

221. A 16-year-old girl comes to your office complaining of blood in her urine. She is asymptomatic, and not menstruating. Urinalysis reveals grossly pink urine, but urine dipstick is negative for blood. Which of the following foods is the likely cause?

a. Spinach
b. Strawberries
c. Raspberries
d. Beets
e. Carrots

222. A 65-year-old African American man is seeing you because he has had blood in his urine for 1 day. On further questioning, you find that the blood appears at the end of micturition, and is not associated with pain, frequency, urgency, or other symptoms. Of the following, which is the most likely cause of his hematuria?

a. Urethral cancer
b. Renal cancer
c. Prostate cancer
d. Urolithiasis
e. Urethral trauma

223. You are seeing a 14-year-old boy who reports seeing blood in his urine. He is currently asymptomatic. On urinalysis, he has more than 10 red blood cells per high-powered field, he has red cell casts, and his creatitine is 2.3 (H). What is the next step in the evaluation?

a. Intravenous pyelography
b. Renal ultrasound
c. Cystoscopy
d. Noncontrast helical CT
e. Antistreptolysin O titer

224. You are evaluating a 35-year-old man with hematuria. His urinalysis does not reveal casts or protein, but does show moderate blood. His urine culture is negative, as is his intravenous pyelogram, and he has a normal creatinine. Which of the following is most appropriate in this case?

a. Reassurance and periodic monitoring
b. Renal ultrasound
c. Cystoscopy
d. ASO titer
e. Renal biopsy

225. A daycare worker presents to your office after turning "yellow." She reports feeling feverish and fatigued, and describes right upper quadrant abdominal pain and nausea. On examination, her skin tone, conjunctivae, and mucous membranes are yellow-tinged. Serologies indicate acute hepatitis A infection. Which of the following is true about this infection?

a. She is most infectious while she is jaundiced
b. Fecal shedding of the virus continues until liver enzymes have normalized
c. Complete recovery is the norm
d. Relapses are common
e. This infection can lead to chronic infection

226. A patient is seeing you in follow up after being hospitalized for acute hepatitis. He is concerned about his risk for hepatocellular carcinoma. Which form of viral hepatitis is associated with a clearly increased risk of hepatocellular carcinoma?

a. Hepatitis A virus
b. Hepatitis B virus
c. Hepatitis C virus
d. Hepatitis D virus
e. Hepatitis E virus

227. You are examining a newborn whose mother has a positive screen for hepatitis B surface antigen. Which of the following is true regarding this situation?

a. When acquired early in life, the large majority of those infected with hepatitis B will have chronic disease
b. If the child has a normal immune system, his likelihood of developing chronic disease is small
c. A higher percentage of adults infected with hepatitis B will develop chronic disease as compared with children
d. A high percentage of children acutely infected will develop fulminant liver disease
e. When Hepatitis B is transmitted perinatally, the child generally develops the typical symptoms of acute hepatitis

228. One of your patients had unprotected intercourse with a partner later found to have chronic hepatitis B. In testing your patient, which of the following serologic markers would be the first to appear?

a. Hepatitis B surface antigen
b. Hepatitis B core antigen
c. The IgM to the core protein (IgM anti-HBc)
d. Hepatitis B e antigen
e. The IgM to Hepatitis B e antigen

229. You are talking with a patient who recently found out that a coworker has Hepatitis C. Which of the following is true about hepatitis C?

a. The hepatitis C virus is found in blood
b. The hepatitis C virus is found in semen
c. The hepatitis C virus is found in vaginal secretions
d. The hepatitis C virus is found in breast milk
e. The hepatitis C virus is found in saliva

230. You are following a patient after an acute hepatitis B infection. His serologies are shown below:

- HBsAg: Positive
- HBeAg: Positive
- IgM anti-HBc: Negative
- IgG anti-HBc: Positive
- Anti-HBs: Negative
- Anti-HBe: Negative
- HBV-DNA: Positive

Which term best describes his disease status?

a. Acute infection, early phase
b. Acute infection, recovery phase
c. Chronic infection, replicating virus
d. Chronic infection, nonreplicating virus
e. Previous exposure with immunity

231. You check serologies on a patient exposed to hepatitis B. His serologies are shown below:

- HBsAg: Negative
- HBeAg: Negative
- IgM anti-HBc: Negative
- IgG anti-HBc: Negative
- Anti-HBs: Positive
- Anti-HBe: Negative
- HBV-DNA: Negative

Which term best describes his disease status?

a. Acute infection, early phase
b. Acute infection, window phase
c. Acute infection, recovery phase
d. Previous exposure with immunity
e. Vaccination

232. You are following a patient after an acute hepatitis B infection. His serologies are shown below:

- HBsAg: Positive
- HBeAg: Positive
- IgM anti-HBc: Positive
- IgG anti-HBc: Negative
- Anti-HBs: Negative
- Anti-HBe: Negative
- HBV-DNA: Positive

Which term best describes his disease status?

a. Acute infection, early phase
b. Acute infection, recovery phase
c. Chronic infection, replicating virus
d. Chronic infection, nonreplicating virus
e. Previous exposure with immunity

233. A 59-year-old woman is discussing urinary symptoms with you. She describes mild loss of urine with sneezing, coughing, and laughing. Which of the following is a normal age-related phenomenon that may predispose elderly patients to incontinence?

a. The frequency of involuntary bladder contractions decreases with age (potentially leading to overflow incontinence)
b. Total bladder capacity decreases with age (potentially leading to urge incontinence)
c. Total bladder contractility increases with age (potentially leading to stress incontinence)
d. Elderly patients excrete a larger percentage of fluid earlier in the day (potentially leading to overflow incontinence)
e. Elderly women have urogenital atrophy due to decreased estrogen, and thus have increased sensitivity of the internal urethral sphincter (potentially leading to urge incontinence)

234. You are evaluating a 74-year-old woman for the recent onset of incontinence. She has diabetes, controlled by diet but with recently increasing sugars, and hypertension, controlled with a combination of lisinopril/hydrochlorothiazide. She has complained of constipation recently, and has not had a bowel movement for 3 days. Microscopic analysis of her urine is positive for bacteria, but she does not report dysuria, urgency, or frequency. Which of the following is least likely to be a secondary cause for her incontinence?

a. Hyperglycemia
b. Diuretic use
c. Constipation
d. Bacteruria
e. Postmenopausal state

235. You are caring for a 42-year-old woman complaining of incontinence. She reports often having a strong, often immediate need to void, followed by an involuntary loss of urine. She says her symptoms develop so suddenly, she often urinates while trying to get to the bathroom. Which of the following best describes the type of incontinence she is experiencing?

a. Functional incontinence
b. Senile incontinence
c. Urge incontinence
d. Stress incontinence
e. Overflow incontinence

236. You are performing a review of systems on a 36-year-old mother of five. She carried all children to term, and had five successful vaginal deliveries. She reports leakage of a small amount of urine at the same time as she sneezes. Recently, it also occurs with exercise. Which of the following best describes the type of incontinence she is experiencing?

a. Functional incontinence
b. Senile incontinence
c. Urge incontinence
d. Stress incontinence
e. Overflow incontinence

237. One of your patients, a 70-year-old man, complains of frequently dribbling urine throughout the day. On occasion, he loses a large amount of urine without warning. He is otherwise healthy and takes no other medications. Based on his profile and symptoms, what term best describes his symptoms?

a. Functional incontinence
b. Senile incontinence
c. Urge incontinence
d. Stress incontinence
e. Overflow incontinence

238. You are working up a 66-year-old man with incontinence. You have ruled out secondary causes, and choose to measure the urine left in his bladder after urinating. You calculate this "postvoid" residual as 250 mL. Which of the following is true?

a. Postvoid residual measurement has no place in the workup of incontinence
b. This amount is below what is expected, and leads one to suspect urge incontinence
c. This amount is about average, and is not helpful in determining this patient's type of incontinence
d. This amount is more than average, but is not helpful in determining this patient's type of incontinence
e. This amount is more than average, and would lead one to suspect overflow incontinence

239. You are treating a 40-year-old woman for incontinence. She'd prefer not to use medications, and would like to try pelvic floor strengthening (Kegel) exercises. Which of the following types of incontinence has shown the best response to pelvic floor strengthening exercises?

a. Functional incontinence
b. Stress incontinence
c. Urge incontinence
d. Overflow incontinence
e. Mixed incontinence

240. One of your patients has tried and failed behavioral therapy for incontinence. He describes a strong urge to urinate, followed by involuntary loss of urine. Which of the following would be the best medication for him to use?

a. Oxybutynin (Ditropan)
b. Pseudoephedrine (Sudafed)
c. Trimethoprim-sulfamethoxazole (Bactrim, Septra)
d. Finasteride (Proscar)
e. Terazosin (Hytrin)

241. You are evaluating a 14-year-old female patient whose mother brought her in for evaluation. Despite the fact that all of her friends have started menstruating, the daughter has not. On examination, she has no breast development, no axillary or pubic hair, and her pelvic examination reveals normal appearing anatomy. She has not lost weight recently and is not excessively thin. What is the most likely cause of her primary amenorrhea?

a. Gonadal dysgenesis
b. Hypothalamic failure
c. Pituitary failure
d. Polycystic ovarian syndrome
e. Constitutional delay of puberty

242. You are seeing a 17-year-old patient who began menstruating at age 14, and has been relatively regular since age 15. She made an appointment to be seen today because she stopped having periods 2 months ago. She denies sexual activity. What is the most common cause of secondary amenorrhea?

a. Polycystic ovarian syndrome
b. Functional hypothalamic amenorrhea
c. Pregnancy
d. Hypothyroidism
e. Hyperprolactinemia

243. A 16-year-old woman comes to your office complaining of unpredictable menstrual periods. She began her periods at age 14, and they have never been predictable. She denies sexual activity in her lifetime, has no systemic illness, uses no medications regularly, and her physical examination is normal. What is her most likely diagnosis?

a. Pregnancy
b. Ovulatory bleeding
c. Anovulatory bleeding
d. Uterine leiomyoma
e. Endometrial polyposis

244. A healthy 60-year-old woman is seeing you to evaluate vaginal bleeding. She has not had a menstrual period for approximately 7 years, but 3 months ago noted occasional pink spotting. Since then, it has increased in amount and has become almost continuous. She is currently sexually active with her husband. On examination, she appears well, her pelvic examination is normal, and screens for sexually transmitted infections are negative. What would be your next step?

a. Pelvic ultrasound to evaluate for fibroids
b. Pelvic CT scan to evaluate for pelvic tumor
c. Laparoscopy to evaluate for endometriosis
d. Endometrial biopsy
e. Begin hormone replacement therapy to regulate bleeding

245. You are considering treatment for a 19-year-old female patient with primary dysmenorrhea. What should be your first-line therapy?

a. Use of NSAIDs during menses
b. Use of NSAIDs daily
c. Use of opiates during menses
d. Use of a selective serotonin reuptake inhibitor (SSRI) daily
e. Use of combined oral contraceptive pills daily

246. You are evaluating a 16-year-old who has not menstruated yet. She appears short in stature. Which of the following is the most likely genetic diagnosis?

a. Turner's syndrome
b. Fragile X syndrome
c. Down syndrome
d. Testicular feminization syndrome
e. Factor V Leiden deficiency

247. You are evaluating a 32-year-old woman complaining of amenorrhea. She has mild hypertension, hypothyroidism, gastroesophageal reflux disease, and depression. On evaluation, her prolactin level was found to be 89 ng/mL (H). Which of the following medications would be most likely to cause the elevated prolactin level?

a. Proton pump inhibitors
b. Selective serotonin reuptake inhibitors
c. Thiazide diuretics
d. ACE inhibitors
e. Thyroid hormone replacement

248. You are evaluating 32-year-old woman who has not menstruated in 4 months. She has a long history of irregular menstrual periods, but has never gone this long without a period in the past. She is not pregnant, her laboratory evaluation is normal, and you decide to perform a progestin challenge test. The week after she takes 10 mg of medroxyprogesterone acetate (Provera) for 7 days, she reports having a period. Which of the following is the most likely cause of her amenorrhea?

a. Premature ovarian failure
b. Ovarian neoplasm
c. Turner's syndrome
d. Asherman's syndrome
e. Polycystic ovarian syndrome

249. During the workup of amenorrhea in a 44-year-old woman, you discover her testosterone levels are elevated (322 ng/dL) and her DHEA-S levels are also elevated (9 mg/dL). Which of the following would be appropriate in this setting?

a. CT scanning of the adrenal glands
b. Hysteroscopy
c. Hysterosalpingogram
d. MRI of the brain
e. Karyotyping

250. You are evaluating a 16-year-old girl who has never menstruated. She has normal secondary sexual characteristics, and her laboratory evaluation is negative. She has no withdrawal bleeding after a progestin challenge, and you choose to perform an estrogen-progestin challenge. She has no withdrawal bleeding after that challenge as well. Which of the following is the most likely reason for her amenorrhea?

a. An outflow tract obstruction
b. Hypergonadotropic amenorrhea
c. Hypogonadotropic amenorrhea
d. Polycystic ovarian syndrome
e. Pituitary adenoma

251. You are seeing a 24-year-old woman complaining of dysmenorrhea. She has always had painful periods, but lately they seem to be worsening. Her physical examination, including pelvic examination, is normal. She is not currently sexually active. Which of the following is the most appropriate next step in the workup?

a. No further workup is needed
b. Gonorrhea and Chlamydia cultures
c. Pelvic ultrasound
d. Hysterosalpingography
e. Laparoscopy

252. You are evaluating an 18-year-old college student complaining of painful menstrual periods. She reports that she began menstruating at age 14. Since that time, her periods have always been associated with pain. The pain begins just prior to her period starting, and lasts for up to 3 days. She has associated nausea, fatigue, and headache. Which of the following is the most likely diagnosis?

a. Primary dysmenorrhea
b. Endometriosis
c. Leiomyoma
d. Adenomyosis
e. Ovarian cysts

253. You are evaluating a 20-year-old with dysmenorrhea. Her history and physical examination are normal, and you choose to treat her with a trial of oral contraceptives. How do oral contraceptives work to treat dysmenorrhea?

a. Suppressing of prostaglandin synthesis
b. Suppressing of prostaglandin release
c. Causing endometrial hyperplasia
d. Increasing vasoconstriction in the uterus
e. Directly decreasing uterine resting tone

254. You are caring for a 70-year-old hospitalized male who is currently 1 day out from a carotid endarterectomy. You are called to the floor at 3:00 a.m. because the patient removed his peripheral IV and is demanding to go home. Reviewing his chart, you see he has a history of hypertension and hyperlipidemia, both of which are well controlled with medication. He is working part-time as an auto mechanic, and lives at home with his wife. On evaluation, he is agitated but responds to questions, oriented to person only, and denies chest pain, palpitations, shortness of breath, dizziness, or other problems. Of the following, which characteristic points to delirium instead of dementia in this case?

a. The acute onset of his symptoms
b. The fact that he is disoriented to time and place
c. His history of hypertension
d. The fact that he is responsive to questions
e. The fact that this happened in the early morning hours

255. You are in the emergency room caring for a 47-year-old man who was brought in by his wife who states that he had an acute onset of confusion. His past medical history is unremarkable, without evidence of drug or alcohol use. On examination, you find his blood pressure to be 210/130, his pulse to be 97, and his respirations to be 20 per minute. His temperature is 98.4°F. Strength, sensation, and gait are normal. He has no tremor. What would you expect to find on ophthalmologic examination?

a. Pinpoint pupils
b. Dilated pupils
c. Papilledema
d. 6th cranial nerve palsy
e. Anisocoria of 1 mm

256. You are evaluating a homeless person in the emergency department who is displaying a hyperalert confusion. Withdrawal of which of the following substances is most likely to cause this state?

a. Levothyroxine
b. Fluoxetine
c. Oxycodone/acetaminophen
d. Alcohol
e. Amphetamine

257. You receive a telephone call from the roommate of an 18-year-old college freshman who is your patient. The roommate states the patient complained of a headache, aches, and a low-grade fever throughout the day. The patient went to take a nap 20 minutes ago, and is now difficult to arouse. Which of the following tests would be most likely to reveal the diagnosis?

a. Urinalysis
b. Complete blood count
c. Toxicology screen
d. Pregnancy test
e. Lumbar puncture

258. You are seeing a 70-year-old woman who was brought to the office by her daughter. The daughter says she is worried, because her mother seems more forgetful lately. She has a 20-year history of type 2 diabetes, controlled with glucophage. On examination, she is mildly hypertensive with otherwise normal vital signs. She is oriented to time, place, and person. She is unable to complete "serial sevens" on the mini-mental status examination. Which of the following features would be more consistent with dementia as opposed to delirium?

a. Her mild hypertension
b. Her long history of diabetes
c. Her current level of consciousness
d. The inability to complete serial sevens
e. The recent onset of her symptoms

259. You are discussing symptoms of nausea and vomiting with a 52-year-old female patient with longstanding type 2 diabetes mellitus. She reports chronic symptoms that become worse after eating. She will occasionally vomit 1 or 2 hours after eating, and the food that comes up is undigested. On examination, she has not lost weight, and is not showing signs of clinical dehydration. What is the best treatment for her condition?

a. An anticholinergic medication, like scopolamine (Transderm Scop)
b. An antihistamine, like promethazine (Phenergan)
c. A benzamide, like metoclopramide (Reglan)
d. A cannabinoid, like dronabinol (Marinol)
e. A phenothiazine, like chlorpromazine (Thorazine)

260. You are evaluating a 63-year-old man who complains of abdominal pain, distension, nausea, and vomiting. It began rather suddenly this morning, though he has had mild pain for several days. His past history is significant for a partial sigmoid resection for diverticulosis and an appendectomy at age 23. On examination, he is afebrile, his mucous membranes are dry, but he has no orthostatic symptoms. His abdomen is distended and diffusely tender, and his bowel sounds are hyperactive. Which of the following is the most likely cause of his nausea and vomiting?

a. Gastroenteritis
b. Ileus
c. Obstruction
d. Diverticulosis
e. Diverticulitis

261. You are seeing a 12-year-old girl for nausea and vomiting. She was diagnosed as having viral gastroenteritis in the emergency department more than 6 weeks ago, but since that time has had difficulty keeping food down. She states that whenever she eats, she gets nauseated and vomits within 10–30 minutes. She has been using antiemetics to control her symptoms, but they do not work consistently. She has always done well in school, and denies social stressors. Her medical history is unremarkable, but she was treated for depression last year. On examination, she is well-nourished, interactive and in no distress with no signs of dehydration. Her weight is 147 lb—5 lb less than at her well examination 6 months ago—and her height is 5 ft. What is the most likely cause of her symptoms?

a. Chronic gastroenteritis
b. Psychogenic vomiting
c. Anorexia nervosa
d. Bulimia nervosa
e. Central nervous system malignancy

262. You are seeing a 6-year-old boy with nausea and vomiting. His symptoms began acutely last evening, starting with malaise, headache, low-grade fever, body aches, and diarrhea. On examination, he has dry mucous membranes, but no orthostatic symptoms. He has diffuse mild abdominal pain without rebound or involuntary guarding. What is the best treatment for his condition?

a. Nothing by mouth until his symptoms improve
b. Oral rehydration with clear liquids, advancing the diet as tolerated
c. Intravenous rehydration, advancing to oral as tolerated

d. Antiemetics, given intravenously or intramuscularly
e. Trimethoprim/sulfamethoxazole therapy

263. You are seeing a 44-year-old woman with hypertension controlled with lisinopril, who presents with severe nausea and vomiting. She reports having months of occasional right upper quadrant pain, usually after eating out with her husband, that resolves within a couple of hours. Over the last 24 hours, her symptoms have been severe, and she is unable to eat or drink without vomiting. Her pain is significant, radiates to her back, and is better when she leans forward. On laboratory evaluation, her amylase is elevated, and her alanine aminotransferase (ALT) is elevated. Which of the following would be the best approach to avoid recurrent problems in her case?

a. Discontinue lisinopril
b. Avoid calcium in the diet
c. Work with the patient to remain sober
d. Remove the patient's gallbladder
e. Use medication to lower the patient's triglyceride level

264. You are evaluating a 38-year-old man who is complaining of nausea and vomiting. He reports that he is nauseated before breakfast, and the vomiting is described as "projectile." The symptoms improve throughout the day. It is also associated with some headache and subjective dizziness. Of the following, which is the most likely diagnosis?

a. Gastroparesis
b. Cholelithiasis
c. Pancreatitis
d. A vestibular disorder
e. A brain tumor

265. You are evaluating a 45-year-old obese woman who is complaining of nausea. Occasionally, she vomits what appears to be undigested food. Her symptoms occur an hour or two after eating meals, and she denies any pain. What is the most likely diagnosis?

a. Gastroparesis
b. Cholelithiasis
c. Pancreatitis
d. A vestibular disorder
e. A brain tumor

266. A new mother brings her infant to see you to discuss his vomiting. He is 4 weeks old, and is exclusively breast-fed. He vomits with every meal. On examination, his abdomen is distended with normal bowel sounds, and he appears dehydrated. He has lost 4 oz since his visit with you 2 weeks ago. What is the most likely diagnosis?

a. Allergy to breast milk
b. Normal gastroesophageal reflux
c. Pyloric stenosis
d. Intussesception
e. Small bowel obstruction

267. You are evaluating a 31 year-old man with the acute onset of nausea and vomiting. It is associated with significant epigastric pain that radiates to the back and occurs after eating any type of food. It is somewhat better if he does not eat at all. Which of the following tests is most likely to be abnormal in this case?

a. Complete blood count
b. Amylase and lipase
c. Hemoccult testing of the stool
d. Abdominal x-rays
e. Upper endoscopy

268. You are evaluating a 44-year-old woman with the acute onset of nausea and vomiting. It is associated with pain, and occurs after eating a fatty meal. Which of the following tests is most likely to be abnormal in this case?

a. Amylase and lipase
b. Hemoccult testing of the stool
c. Abdominal x-rays
d. Ultrasound
e. Upper endoscopy

269. You are treating a 26-year-old woman for nausea. Which of the following antiemetics is most likely to cause extrapyramidal reactions in the patient?

a. Trimethobenzamide (Tigan)
b. Prochlorperazine (Compazine)
c. Promethazine (Phenergan)
d. Metoclopramide (Reglan)
e. Ondansetron (Zofran)

270. You are evaluating a 33-year-old woman complaining of palpitations. Which of the following characteristics, if present, increase the likelihood that the symptoms are cardiac in etiology?

a. The fact that the patient is female
b. The fact that the patient has a sister with similar symptoms
c. Her description of the symptoms as an "irregular heartbeat"
d. The fact that her father has a history of heart disease
e. The fact that the episodes last less than 1 minute

271. You are seeing a hypertensive 56-year-old woman who is complaining of a "fluttering in her chest." She describes a rapid heart rate, and to her it seems irregular. She is otherwise well, and denies shortness of breath, lightheadedness pedal edema or other acute symptoms. On examination, her pulse rate is rapid and irregular. Which of the following is her most likely diagnosis?

a. Atrial fibrillation
b. Paroxysmal supraventricular tachycardia (PSVT)
c. Stable ventricular tachycardia
d. Stimulant abuse
e. Hyperthyroidism

272. You are seeing a 32-year-old otherwise healthy woman who is complaining of palpitations. She describes the sensation as a "flip flop" in her chest. They only last an instant, and are not associated with lightheadedness or other symptoms. She denies other symptoms. Which of the following is the most likely etiology of her complaint?

a. Atrial fibrillation
b. PSVT
c. Ventricular premature beats
d. Stimulant abuse
e. Hyperthyroidism

273. You are seeing a 22-year-old African American man who is complaining of an irregular heartbeat. He says that when he is exercising, he can feel his heartbeat, and it is more than what he would expect with exertion. It is associated with some lightheadedness and shortness of breath. On examination, his heart has a regular rate and rhythm, but you note a harsh holosystolic murmur along the left sternal border. It seems to increase with Valsalva's maneuver. Which of the following is the most likely cause of his symptoms?

a. Mitral valve prolapse
b. Hypertrophic obstructive cardiomyopathy
c. Dilated cardiomyopathy
d. Atrial fibrillation
e. CHF

274. You are seeing a 26-year-old woman who is complaining of "skipping heartbeats." She uses caffeine daily, but denies other stimulants. The rest of her history is completely normal, as is her physical examination. In the office, her 12-lead ECG is also normal. Her electrolytes and CBC comes back normal, as does her thyroid stimulating hormone. Which of the following is the next step in her workup?

a. Reassure her and continue observation
b. Perform ambulatory ECG monitoring (a 24-Holter monitor, or a continuous loop event recorder)
c. Electrophysiology consultation
d. Stress testing
e. Echocardiography

275. You are evaluating a 23-year-old African American swimmer who is complaining of episodes of symptomatic rapid heart beating. Twice during swim practice, he develops a sensation that his heart is racing. When he measures his heart rate, he finds it to be between 140–160 beats per minute. The first episode lasted approximately 4 minutes, and the second lasted more than 10 minutes. He denies lightheadedness or other symptoms during the events. Limited laboratory evaluation and ECG are normal. Which of the following is the next step in the evaluation?

a. Reassure and continue observation
b. Ambulatory ECG monitoring
c. Consultation with an electrophysiologist
d. Stress testing
e. Echocardiography

276. You are seeing a man complaining of symptomatic palpitations. His ECG is shown below:

(Reproduced, with permission, from Ferry D. Basic Electrocardiography in Ten Days, 1st ed. New York: McGraw-Hill, 2001: 177.)

What is the likely diagnosis?

a. Sinus tachycardia
b. Supraventricular tachycardia
c. Wolff-Parkinson-White syndrome
d. Ventricular tachycardia
e. Premature atrial contractions

277. You are caring for a 23-year-old woman complaining of pelvic pain. She reports one-sided pain that is diffuse and dull, but occasionally sharp. Menses have been normal. She denies fever. Her pelvic examination is normal with the exception of a smooth mobile adnexal mass on the right side. What is the most likely cause of the pain?

a. Pelvic inflammatory disease
b. Ectopic pregnancy
c. Ovarian cyst
d. Uterine leiomyoma
e. Appendicitis

278. You are caring for a 21-year-old woman complaining of pelvic pain. She reports a gradual onset of bilateral pain associated with fever, vaginal discharge, and mild dysuria. Her pelvic examination demonstrates uterine, adnexal, and cervical motion tenderness. What is the most likely cause of the pain?

a. Pelvic inflammatory disease
b. Ectopic pregnancy
c. Ovarian cyst
d. Uterine leiomyoma
e. Appendicitis

279. You are caring for a 27-year-old woman complaining of pelvic pain. She reports localized pain on the left side that has increased in severity over the last 2 days. She also reports amenorrhea and nausea. On examination, you note a tender adnexal mass on the left. What is the likely cause?

a. Pelvic inflammatory disease
b. Ectopic pregnancy
c. Ovarian cyst
d. Uterine leiomyoma
e. Appendicitis

280. You are evaluating a 33-year-old woman with chronic pelvic pain. She reports cyclic pain, generally during the premenstrual period and during her menses. She has been trying to conceive for 15 months without success. Her pelvic examination is normal. Which of the following tests would be most helpful in determining the cause of her pain?

a. Complete blood cell count
b. Erythrocyte sedimentation rate
c. CA-125 levels
d. Transvaginal pelvic ultrasound
e. Magnetic resonance imaging

281. You are evaluating a 13-year-old girl with pelvic pain. She is not sexually active, and you do not have suspicion of abuse. On pelvic examination, you confirm that she has never been sexually active, but feel an ovarian mass on the right side. Which of the following approaches is most appropriate in this case?

a. Reassurance and use of NSAIDs for pain control
b. Reassurance and repeat pelvic examination in 6–8 weeks
c. Transvaginal pelvic ultrasound
d. CT scanning of the abdomen and pelvis
e. MRI evaluation of the pelvis

282. You are evaluating a 18-year-old male with a sore throat. It has been present for 3 days, and is associated with fever, aches, and fatigue. On examination, he has an exudative pharyngitis, soft palate petechiae, and posterior cervical adenopathy. Which of the following is the most likely diagnosis?

a. Group A streptococcal infection
b. Group A streptococcal colonization
c. *Corynebacterium diphtheriae* infection
d. Gonorrhea infection of the throat
e. Epstein-Barr virus infection

283. A 7-year-old boy comes to see you for a sore throat. He reports fevers, chills, myalgias, and pain on swallowing. On examination, you note anterior adenopathy, erythematous tonsils, and uveal edema. He has no drug allergies. Which of the following would be the best treatment for his condition?

a. Symptomatic care
b. Antiviral therapy
c. Doxycycline (Vibramycin)
d. Amoxicillin (Amoxil)
e. Erythromycin (Emycin)

284. You are treating a 16-year-old girl with a sore throat. She denies runny nose or cough, but does report fevers and myalgia. On examination, she has an exudative pharyngitis, and posterior cervical adenopathy. Her rapid streptococcal antigen is positive. You treat her with penicillin, and she develops a diffuse maculopapular rash. What is the most likely diagnosis?

a. Scarlet fever
b. Infectious mononucleosis
c. Viral exanthem
d. Pityriasis rosea
e. Tinea versicolor

285. An 8-year-old patient has a positive group A streptococcal throat culture whether symptomatic or not. You have determined that he is a streptococcal carrier. Assuming that the patient has no allergies, what is the best therapeutic option in this patient?

a. Penicillin (PenVK)
b. Amoxicillin (Amoxil), using the usual dose
c. Amoxicillin (Amoxil), using high dosages
d. Erythromycin (Emycin)
e. Clindamycin (Cleocin)

286. You are treating a 16-year-old patient with a sore throat. She has had 3 days of symptoms, and does not have nasal congestion or cough. She also reports laryngitis. On examination, she has an erythematous pharynx without exudate. Which of the following is the most appropriate therapy based on the symptoms described?

a. Supportive care
b. Penicillin (PenVK)
c. Amoxicillin (Amoxil)
d. Erythromycin (Emycin)
e. Clindamycin (Cleocin)

287. You are caring for a teen with fairly severe acne. Which of the following has been shown to play a role in the development of acne?

a. Stress
b. Dirty skin
c. Chocolate
d. Increased greasy foods in the diet
e. Oily hair on the forehead

288. One of your patients is concerned about facial acne. He has both inflammatory and comedonal acne (see picture below), and you would rate it as moderate in severity. Which of the following would be the best approach to treating his acne?

(Reproduced, with permission, from Wolff K, Johnson RA, Suurmond D. Fitzpatrick's Color Atlas and Synopsis of Clinical Dermatology, 5th ed. New York: McGraw-Hill, 2005: 5.)

a. A topical retinoid such as tretinoin (Retin-A)
b. A topical antibiotic such as erythromycin or clindamycin (Em-gel or Cleocin)
c. An oral antibiotic such as cephalexin (Keflex)
d. An oral contraceptive
e. A mid-potency nonfluorinated topical steroid

289. You are treating a 16-year-old girl who is complaining of severe nodular acne. She has tried and failed topical retinoids and oral antibiotics, and you are considering using isotretinoin (Accutane). Which of the following is a significant side effect that warrants discontinuing the medication?

a. Depression
b. Worsening of acne
c. Dry skin
d. Joint aches
e. Pregnancy

290. You are caring for a 34-year-old woman who complains of a chronic "blush" around her cheeks and nose. Her picture is below:

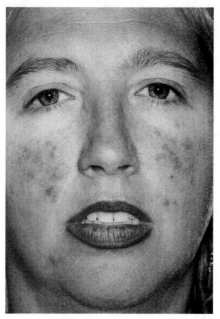

(Reproduced, with permission, from Wolff K, Johnson RA, Suurmond D. Fitzpatrick's Color Atlas and Synopsis of Clinical Dermatology, 5th ed. New York: McGraw-Hill, 2005: 9.)

Which of the following is true of this condition?

a. It has a pathogenesis similar to acne vulgaris
b. About 50% of patients with this condition also have eye involvement
c. Topical corticosteroids are the treatment of choice
d. Oral therapy with tetracyclines should be reserved as a last resort
e. Treatment should be aimed at reducing colonization of *Propionibacterium acnes*

291. A patient comes to you with concerns about a nodule he has had on the side of his nose for several months. The nodule is shown below:

(Reproduced, with permission, from Wolff K, Johnson RA, Suurmond D. Fitzpatrick's Color Atlas and Synopsis of Clinical Dermatology, 5th ed. New York: McGraw-Hill, 2005: 283.)

What is the most likely diagnosis?

a. Verruca vulgaris
b. Molluscum contagiosum
c. Nodular basal cell carcinoma
d. Squamous cell carcinoma
e. Cutaneous T-cell lymphoma

292. You are caring for a 28-year-old man who presents with a rash. A picture of his rash is shown below:

(Reproduced, with permission, from Wolff K, Johnson RA, Suurmond D. Fitzpatrick's Color Atlas and Synopsis of Clinical Dermatology, 5th ed. New York: McGraw-Hill, 2005: 59.)

He also has fingernail changes shown below:

(Reproduced, with permission, from Wolff K, Johnson RA, Suurmond D. Fitzpatrick's Color Atlas and Synopsis of Clinical Dermatology, 5th ed. New York: McGraw-Hill, 2005: 993.)

What is the most commonly prescribed therapeutic agent for his rash?

a. Oral Penicillin
b. Topical erythromycin
c. Topical pimecrolimus (Elidel)
d. Vitamin A
e. Topical corticosteroids

293. You are discussing therapy with a patient who has recently been diagnosed with psoriasis. He is interested in trying calcipotriene (Dovonex). Which of the following best describes its mechanism of action?

a. It is a fatty-acid based moisturizer
b. It induces epidermal differentiation and inhibits keratinocyte proliferation
c. It binds to retinoic acid receptors in the skin, normalizing the epidermal proliferation
d. It is a topical immunomodulator
e. It is a topical keratolytic

294. You are talking with a 24-year-old man who reports an outbreak of a mildly pruritic rash. The rash initially began with a large pink patch on his chest, to the left of his sternum breast. About a week later, he noted a more generalized eruption. The rash is shown below:

(Reproduced, with permission, from Wolff K, Johnson RA, Suurmond D. Fitzpatrick's Color Atlas and Synopsis of Clinical Dermatology, *5th ed. New York: McGraw-Hill, 2005: 119.)*

What treatment is indicated?

a. Antihistamines
b. Antibiotics
c. Antivirals
d. Antifungals
e. Cyclosporine

295. You are seeing a young child whose mother brings him in with a rash. It developed on his upper lip underneath his nose. He has had cold symptoms with a runny nose recently. His picture is shown below:

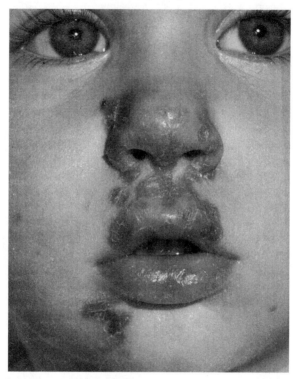

(Reproduced, with permission, from Wolff K, Johnson RA, Suurmond D. Fitzpatrick's Color Atlas and Synopsis of Clinical Dermatology, 5th ed. New York: McGraw-Hill, 2005: 589.)

What is the most likely cause of this rash?

a. Infection with group A beta-hemolytic streptococci
b. Infection with *S. aureus*
c. Infection with an enterococcus species
d. Infection with *H. influenzae*
e. Infection with a pseudomonas species

296. After returning from a ski trip in the mountains, your 35-year-old patient complains of a rash for 2 days. He has multiple eythematous pustules over his legs, arms, and chest. They are not pruritic, and do not seem to be spreading. He denies any new soaps, lotions, foods, or medications. He did spend time in a hot tub on the trip. A picture of his rash is shown below:

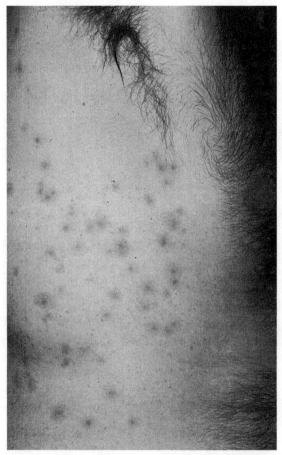

(Reproduced, with permission, from Wolff K, Johnson RA, Suurmond D. Fitzpatrick's Color
Atlas and Synopsis of Clinical Dermatology, 5th ed. New York: McGraw-Hill, 2005: 982.)

Which of the following is the best treatment option for this patient?

a. Reassurance and follow up if no improvement
b. Topical steroid medication
c. Systemic steroid medication
d. Topical antibiotics with activity against streptococcus and staphylococcus
e. Oral antibiotics with activity against *Pseudomonas* species

297. You are seeing a 21-year-old man with a skin infection on his lip. It is the first time he has ever had this type of infection. It began with a burning at the site of the infection, then an eruption of vesicles. The rash is shown below:

(Reproduced, with permission, from Wolff K, Johnson RA, Suurmond D. Fitzpatrick's Color Atlas and Synopsis of Clinical Dermatology, 5th ed. New York: McGraw-Hill, 2005: 803.)

Which of the following is true of this infection?
a. This is a primary infection, and future infections are likely to be more severe
b. Based on the picture shown, distinguishing features indicate it to be a HSV-1 infection
c. Fever, malaise, and adenopathy are likely to be present
d. Triggers for this rash include fever, infection, or exposure to ultraviolet light
e. If the lesions are pustular, antibiotics are indicated

298. Your patient is known to have genital herpes. She has recently had an increase in outbreaks, and is now complaining of symptoms that occur at least every 2 months. Which of the following would be considered an appropriate therapy?
a. Valacyclovir (Valtrex), 1 g twice a day for 10 days with each outbreak
b. Valcyclovir (Valtrex), 2 g in a single dose at the first sign of skin lesion
c. Valcyclovir (Valtrex), 2 g in a single dose at the first sign of the prodrome
d. Valcyclovir (Valtrex), 1 g weekly
e. Valcyclovir (Valtrex), 1 g daily

299. An otherwise healthy 61-year-old male patient complains of a burning sensation on the posterior chest for 24 hours, and subsequent development of the rash shown below:

(Reproduced, with permission, from Wolff K, Johnson RA, Suurmond D. Fitzpatrick's Color Atlas and Synopsis of Clinical Dermatology, *5th ed. New York: McGraw-Hill, 2005: 823.)*

Which of the following is true about treatment for this condition?

a. Antiviral therapy is not indicated if the lesions have been present for more than 72 hours
b. Antiviral therapy decreases the overall duration of pain
c. Treatment with corticosteroids will decrease the likelihood of postherpetic neuralgia
d. Valacyclovir (Valtrex) is the best antiviral treatment choice for this condition
e. Antiviral resistance is common

300. You are seeing a young girl whose mother brings her in for evaluation. She has had 3 days of low-grade fever and runny nose. Today, she awakened with a rash on her cheeks, shown below:

(Reproduced, with permission, from Wolff K, Johnson RA, Suurmond D. Fitzpatrick's Color Atlas and Synopsis of Clinical Dermatology, 5th ed. New York: McGraw-Hill, 2005: 793.)

What is the likely cause of her symptoms?

a. An enterovirus
b. A parvovirus
c. A parainfluenza virus
d. A varicella virus
e. Cytomegalovirus

301. You are seeing a young man who is complaining of a patch of hair loss. He denies pulling the hair, and complains that his scalp is itchy and flakey. His scalp is shown below:

(Reproduced, with permission, from Wolff K, Johnson RA, Suurmond D. Fitzpatrick's Color Atlas and Synopsis of Clinical Dermatology, 5th ed. New York: McGraw-Hill, 2005: 709.)

Which of the following is the most effective treatment?
a. Selenium sulfide lotion, applied daily for 4–8 weeks
b. Ketoconazole (Nizoral) shampoo applied daily for 4–8 weeks
c. Clotrimazole (Lotrimin) cream, twice daily for 4–8 weeks
d. Griseofulvin tablets, daily for 4–8 weeks
e. Fluconazole (Diflucan) tablets, daily for 4–8 weeks

302. You are caring for a 35-year-old woman who works in a daycare. She comes to see you complaining of an itchy rash on her calf. It started as a small pink circular lesion, but is spreading. The rash is shown below:

(Reproduced, with permission, from Wolff K, Johnson RA, Suurmond D. Fitzpatrick's Color Atlas and Synopsis of Clinical Dermatology, 5th ed. New York: McGraw-Hill, 2005: 701.)

Which of the following is the likely diagnosis?

a. Pityriasis rosea
b. Psoriasis
c. Tinea corporis
d. Atopic dermatitis
e. Contact dermatitis

303. A 32-year-old mother of two young children presents to your office for evaluation of her left eye. She reports redness of the white part of her eye, with a watery discharge. She reports mild itching and a sensation as if something is in her eye. She denies a history of allergies, and reports no concurrent allergic symptoms. Examination reveals a palpable preauricular lymph node. Fluorescein staining does not reveal corneal dendrites. What should be the treatment of choice in this case?

a. Antiviral eye drops
b. Antibacterial eye drops
c. Corticosteroid eye drops
d. Combination antibiotic/corticosteroid eye drops
e. Supportive care

304. Which of the following causes of a red eye is a medical emergency and requires immediate ophthalmologic referral?

a. Gonococcal conjunctivitis
b. Chlamydial conjunctivitis
c. Corneal abrasion
d. Sub-conjunctival hemorrhage
e. Blepharitis

305. You are seeing a 26-year-old male patient complaining of a red eye who says, "I think I have pink eye." He reports increased redness, tearing, discharge, photophobia, and pain. Which of his reported symptoms would be more suggestive of something other than conjunctivitis?

a. Redness
b. Tearing
c. Discharge
d. Photophobia
e. Pain

306. You are seeing a 20-year-old college student who reports that her eye became pink over the last 24 hours. She is otherwise healthy and takes no medications except oral contraceptives. She reports redness, irritation, tearing, discharge, and itching. Which of her symptoms are more specific for an allergic etiology for her condition?

a. Use of oral contraceptives
b. Irritation
c. Tearing
d. Discharge
e. Itching

307. You are caring for a 3-year-old boy who goes to daycare while his parents are at work. His mother brought him to see you because the daycare will not take him back until he's had a doctor evaluate his eye symptoms. He developed an acute redness of the left eye, associated with runny nose, cough, and increased irritability. On examination, his eye is red and watery. The discharge is clear, and he has mild eyelid edema. Which of the following is the most common cause for his condition?

a. Coxsackie virus
b. Parainfluenza virus
c. Adenovirus
d. Rhinovirus
e. Herpes virus

308. You are seeing a 32-year-old contact lens wearer who has recently suffered from recurrent conjunctivitis. Which of the following treatments would be best in this situation?

a. Supportive care
b. Ciprofloxacin (Ciloxan) ointment
c. Ploymyxin-trimentoprim (Polytrim) ointment
d. Gentamicin (Garamycin) ointment
e. Immediate ophthalmologic referral

309. You are evaluating a 20-year-old college student who complains of an acute red eye. He complains that his eye is irritated, with significant yellowish discharge. When he wipes his eye, it almost immediately reforms. You confirm this by wiping his eye with a cotton swab. When asked, he also reports dysuria and penile discharge. What is the most appropriate treatment?

a. Supportive care
b. Ciprofloxacin ointment
c. Tobramycin ointment
d. Ceftriaxone (Rocephin) intramuscularly
e. Immediate ophthalmologic referral

310. You have been treating a 43-year-old woman with rheumatoid arthritis for years. You and her rheumatologist have had her illness in relatively good control. She presents to you with a red eye and significant eye pain. She denies trauma. Upon further questioning, she complains of decreased vision and headache. She describes the pain as deep and boring. Her examination reveals diffuse injection of the deeper vessels with minimal discharge. Her pupils react normally. What is her most likely diagnosis?

a. Scleritis
b. Episcleritis
c. Corneal abrasion
d. Acute glaucoma
e. Iritis

311. You are caring for a 32-year-old female smoker with upper respiratory symptoms. She reports congestion, facial pressure, nasal discharge, tooth pain, and headache. Her symptoms have been present for 14 days. Which portion of her history is most commonly used to define clinical rhinosinusitis?

a. Facial pressure
b. Nasal discharge
c. Tooth pain
d. Headache
e. 14-days of illness

312. A 35-year-old man has been struggling with recurrent sinusitis. He develops at least four sinus infections per year, and wonders what he can do to prevent these. You are discussing predisposing factors with him, in an effort to control any present. Which of the following is the most common predisposing condition leading to chronic or recurrent sinusitis?

a. Allergic rhinitis
b. Gastroesophageal reflux disease
c. Cigarette smoking
d. Environmental pollutants
e. Immunodeficiency

313. You are seeing a 21-year-old college student who complains of congestion, headache, sinus pressure and tooth pain for more than 2 weeks. She is otherwise healthy, but feels like she's "having trouble shaking this cold." She has used over the counter decongestants with limited relief. A CT scan of her sinuses demonstrates acute sinusitis. Of those listed, which is the most common organism causing her symptoms?

a. *Moraxella Catarrhalis*
b. *S. aureus*
c. Group A beta hemolytic streptococcal species
d. *Streptococcus pneumoniae*
e. A polymicrobial mixture of many organisms

314. You are caring for a 42-year-old woman with a persistent sinusitis. She first came to see you 3 months ago, was treated with amoxicillin, and improved. She returned 2 months ago, received another course of amoxicillin, and improved again. Last month, her symptoms reoccurred, and you prescribed trimethoprim/sulfamethoxazole. She returns today with continued symptoms. What would be your treatment of choice?

a. A macrolide for 10 days
b. A macrolide for 14–21 days
c. A fluoroquinolone for 10 days
d. A fluoroquinolone for 14–21 days
e. A second or third generation cephalosporin for 10 days

315. You are treating a woman with chronic and recurrent sinusitis. Along with antibiotic therapy directed at the underlying bacterial cause, which of the following has been shown to help break the cycle of recurrent disease?

a. Phenylpropanolamine
b. Pseudoephedrine
c. Topical alpha agonists (Afrin)
d. Topical nasal steroids
e. Echinacea

316. You are seeing a 16-year-old high school football player to discuss a recent injury. Last night, during football practice, he felt an acute numbness and tingling from his neck down to his right hand, "like an electric shock." The inciting event occurred when he was tackled, compressing his head, while his head and neck were flexed toward the right side. The numbness resolved within a few minutes, but he did not continue play. He is seeing you for evaluation and treatment. He currently has normal range of motion, with no neurological deficit or pain. What is the most appropriate next step?

a. Return to play without restriction
b. Immobilization until radiographs can be obtained
c. Immobilization until magnetic resonance imaging can be obtained
d. Obtain an electromyelogram of the right arm before allowing return to play
e. Refer for physical therapy

317. You are working with the team physician at a local high school. One of the football players was hit with his arm extended, causing a left shoulder injury. On examination, he has acromioclavicular (AC) joint swelling, bruising, and pain. X-rays show more than a 50% AC joint separation with a posterior displacement of the clavicle. Which of the following is the best management plan for this injury?

a. Return to play when the pain subsides
b. Immobilization with a sling, and return to play when the pain subsides
c. Immobilization with a sling, and early range of motion exercises with return to play when the pain subsides
d. Reduction under conscious sedation, then immobilization, early range of motion exercises, and return to play when the pain subsides
e. Surgical fixation

318. A 20-year-old college basketball player comes to your office complaining of knee pain. Her symptoms started several weeks ago, but she was able to play through the pain. She reports anterior knee pain, some mild swelling after activity, and significant stiffness and pain after she's been sitting for a long period of time. Examination reveals a positive patellar grind test. Based on her history and examination, which of the following exercises would be most likely to help her symptoms?

a. Patellar tendon stretching
b. Quadriceps stretching
c. Vastus lateralis strengthening
d. Vastus medialis strengthening
e. Hamstring strengthening

319. A patient comes to see you after a skiing accident 6 days ago. He reports twisting his knee during a fall, feeling a "pop," and noting significant immediate swelling. He was able to bear weight immediately, but did not ski for the rest of the trip. His pain is now improved, and he is ambulating, but he says the knee feels unstable. What is the most likely cause of his symptoms?

a. Patellofemoral pain syndrome
b. Anterior cruciate ligament (ACL) tear
c. Posterior cruciate ligament (PCL) tear
d. Meniscal injury
e. Collateral ligament tear

320. One of your patients injured his knee playing soccer. In trying to determine the extent of his injury, you palpate the joint line with one hand and internally/externally rotate while flexing and extending the knee. This maneuver elicits a catch with pain at the joint line. Which of the following knee injuries is most likely?

a. Patellar tendon rupture
b. Patellar fracture
c. ACL tear
d. Meniscal tear
e. Collateral ligament tear

321. You are seeing a 14-year-old girl who hurt her ankle while dancing yesterday. She reports that her ankle "twisted in" causing immediate pain and the inability to bear weight. In the office, she has bruising and tenderness over the anterior talofibular ligament (ATFL) with acute swelling. She is unable to bear weight due to the pain. Which of the following is the most appropriate next step?

a. Obtain x-rays of her ankle
b. Encourage early mobilization
c. Prescribe rest, ice, compression, and elevation
d. Use a NSAID to help with the pain and inflammation
e. Begin physical therapy

322. A 65-year-old male patient comes to your office after a syncopal episode. Which of the following etiologies of syncope has the highest mortality rate associated with it?

a. Vasovagal syncope
b. Situational syncope
c. Cardiac syncope
d. Vertebrobasilar artery insufficiency
e. Subclavian steal syndrome

323. You are seeing a 55-year-old man who presents with syncope. Regardless of the cause, which of the following tests is always indicated in the workup?

a. Complete blood count
b. Thyroid stimulating hormone
c. ECG
d. Holter monitoring
e. Ambulatory loop ECG

324. A 21-year-old generally healthy college student is seeing you in your office after having "passed out" playing basketball. This has never happened before. He has no significant past medical history and takes no medications. On examination, you note a harsh crescendo-decrescendo systolic murmur, heard best at the apex and radiating to the axilla. Which of the following tests is most likely to reveal the etiology of his syncopal episode?

a. An echocardiogram
b. A Holter monitor
c. A long-term ambulatory loop ECG
d. Stress testing
e. Tilt table testing

325. You are caring for a 49-year-old type 2 diabetic woman who presents to you after passing out. The event occurred 1 day ago, while she was walking up steps to her seat at a movie theatre. She reports that she felt breathless, became hot and sweaty, and the next thing she remembers, she was waking up on the floor. Her diabetes has been fairly well controlled with metformin, and her last glycosolated hemoglobin 1 month ago was 7.9%. Her examination is benign, as is her ECG. Which of the following tests would be most likely to reveal the cause of her syncope?

a. Serum glucose
b. Hemoglobin A1C
c. Echocardiogram
d. Stress testing
e. A 24-hour Holter monitor

326. You are evaluating a 28-year-old woman who has had several episodes of passing out. In general, the events are unpredictable, and are not preceded by any prodrome. Her examination has been consistently normal. Initial workup, including a pregnancy test, hematocrit, serum glucose, orthostatic blood pressures, and ECG were normal. She underwent 24-hour Holter monitoring and long-term ambulatory loop ECG evaluation, both of which were negative. Which of the following is the most appropriate next test?

a. Psychiatric evaluation
b. Carotid Dopplers
c. MRI of the brain
d. Stress testing
e. Tilt-table testing

327. You are evaluating a woman who is complaining of vaginal discharge. She reports clear discharge and some vaginal irritation. She has recently become sexually active for the first time again after a divorce 2 years ago. She and her partner use condoms. On examination, she has a reddened, swollen vulva and a clear exudate. She does not douche. Based on this history, which of the following is the most likely cause of her discharge?

a. Contact dermatitis
b. Mycotic disease
c. Trichomoniasis
d. Bacterial vaginosis
e. Chlamydia infection

328. You are evaluating a 20-year-old woman complaining of vaginal discharge. She reports vaginal itch and white discharge. She has no history of vaginal infections in the past, and has never been sexually active. A KOH preparation of the discharge is shown below:

(Reproduced, with permission, from Wolff K, Johnson RA, Suurmond D. Fitzpatrick's Color Atlas and Synopsis of Clinical Dermatology, 5th ed. New York: McGraw-Hill, 2005: 717.)

Which of the following is the best treatment option for this condition?

a. Reassurance that this is a normal variation and that no treatment is necessary
b. Topical azole applications
c. Topical metronidazole
d. Oral clindamycin
e. Doxycycline

329. You are discussing recurrent vaginal discharge with a patient. She has been evaluated three times in the last 6 months, and has had a vaginal candidiasis each time. She has symptom-free intervals, but the infection seems to be recurrent. She is sexually active, takes birth control pills, and denies other complaints or known illnesses. Which of the following is most likely to improve this patient's condition?

a. Test her for diabetes, and control her elevated glucose level
b. Ask her to discontinue her birth control pills
c. Treat her sexual partner
d. Test her for HIV, and begin therapy
e. Ask her to add fiber to her diet

330. You are evaluating a 16-year-old woman who complains of vaginal itching. She has been sexually active with one partner for 4 months. She also reports urinary frequency. On examination, you note yellow-green bubbly discharge with bright red vaginal mucosa and cervical petechiae. What is the saline preparation of the discharge likely to show?

a. Sheets of epithelial cells "studded" with bacteria
b. "Moth-eaten" epithelial cells
c. Motile triangular cells with long tails
d. Many white blood cells
e. Hyphae

331. Your patient describes a recent vaginal discharge. She reports more discharge than usual, and an unusual odor after intercourse with her husband. A KOH preparation of the discharge produces a fishy odor, and a saline preparation is shown below:

(Reproduced, with permission, from Knoop K, Stack L, Storrow A. Atlas of Emergency Medicine, 2nd ed. New York: McGraw-Hill, 2002: 683.)

Of the following, what is the treatment of choice for her condition?

a. Metronidazole
b. Doxycycline
c. Clotrimazole
d. Imiquimod
e. Acyclovir

332. You are caring for an 18-month-old infant, whose mother brings him in for "wheezing." She reports that he has had a runny nose and a slight cough for 2 days, along with a low-grade fever. On examination, he does not appear to be in respiratory distress, but his lung examination does reveal bilateral wheezing. What is the most likely diagnosis?

a. Acute viral respiratory tract infection
b. Pneumonia
c. Bronchiolitis
d. Aspiration
e. Asthma

333. A 61-year-old man comes to see you for shortness of breath. He has a history of hypertension, type 2 diabetes and hyperlipidemia. He quit smoking 4 years ago after a more than 30-pack year history. On physical examination, he is not in respiratory distress, but he has diffuse wheezing in the bilateral lower lobes of his lungs. His cardiac examination demonstrates an S4, and he demonstrates JVD. Which of the following treatments would likely relieve his symptoms?

a. Antibiotic therapy
b. Epinephrine
c. Steroid therapy
d. Diuretics
e. Anticoagulation

334. You are seeing a 26-year-old woman who presents to your office complaining of "wheezing." On further questioning, she reports acute shortness of breath that occurred while she was at work this morning, and her wheezing is associated with pleuritic pain. She is otherwise healthy, only taking oral contraceptives. On examination, she is tachypneic, but not in acute distress. Auscultation of her lungs is normal. What is the most likely cause of her symptoms?

a. Bronchitis
b. Gastroesophageal reflux
c. Pulmonary embolism
d. Asthma
e. Acute allergic reation

335. You are seeing a 23-year-old man for shortness of breath. He has no history of asthma or wheezing, and is otherwise healthy. His lung examination does reveal significant wheezing bilaterally. Which of the following tests is necessary?

a. Observation and treatment
b. Chest x-ray
c. Peak flow testing
d. Pulmonary function tests
e. A complete blood count

336. You are evaluating a 9-month-old child with recurrent wheezing. His mother also reports that he vomits after formula as well. What is the best test to determine the cause of his wheezing?

a. Pulmonary function testing
b. A chest x-ray
c. Upper GI barium swallow
d. Upper endoscopy
e. A 24-hour pH probe

337. You are evaluating a 35-year-old patient with known asthma. He comes to your office complaining of increased shortness of breath despite compliance with his usual asthma regimen. He reports cough, but denies fever or sputum production. His pulmonary examination reveals wheezing bilaterally without crackles or rhonchi. Which of the following is most useful in this setting?

a. Chest x-ray
b. Peak flow testing
c. Pulmonary function testing
d. A complete blood count
e. A nasopharyngral wash

Acute Complaints

Answers

86. The answer is b. (*South-Paul, pp 348–368.*) The first priority when evaluating abdominal pain is to determine whether the pain is acute or chronic. Sudden and/or severe onset of pain should lead the clinician toward an emergent evaluation. Right lower quadrant pain is suspicious for an acute appendicitis, but by itself is not specific enough to warrant an emergent workup. A "gnawing" sensation is often described with ulcer disease, while pain that worsens after eating is associated with many conditions—pancreatitis, gallbladder disease, or even reflux. In the absence of hemodynamic instability, those causes are less likely to warrant emergent workup. Emesis with pain is not enough, by itself, to warrant emergent workup.

87. The answer is c. (*South-Paul, pp 348–368.*) The location and radiation of pain is often helpful in determining the cause of abdominal pain. Pain from an acute appendicitis usually starts in the periumbilical region before moving to the right lower quadrant. Pancreatitis generally settles in the mid-epigastric region with radiation to the back. Gallbladder pain is typically in the epigastric or right upper quadrant and radiates to the scapula. Esophageal spasm is often referred higher in the chest. GERD is midepigastric and generally does not radiate.

88. The answer is b. (*South-Paul, pp 348–368.*) Advanced age can change the presentation and perception of abdominal pain. In fact, studies estimate that there is a 10–20% reduction in the perceived intensity of the pain per decade after age 60. Only 22% of elderly patients with appendicitis present with classic symptoms, making the diagnosis more difficult. Therefore, a high index of suspicion is necessary. Small bowel obstruction and constipation may cause bilateral lower quadrant pain and decreased appetite, but fever indicates something different. IBS is chronic and generally not associated with fever. Pancreatitis is associated with food intolerance but the associated pain is usually in the epigastric region.

89. The answer is c. (*South-Paul, pp 348–368.*) The specific site of tenderness is classic for many sources of abdominal pain. Sudden cessation of inspiratory effort during deep palpation of the right upper quadrant is called "Murphy's sign" and is suggestive of acute cholecystitis. Hepatitis and gallstones may cause right upper quadrant tenderness, but generally do not elicit Murphy's sign. Pain caused by pancreatitis often radiates to the back. Pain from renal calculi often radiates to the shoulder.

90. The answer is c. (*South-Paul, pp 348–368.*) A CT scan of the abdomen and pelvis with and without contrast is usually the most helpful imaging study to confirm a diagnosis, or if not, to dictate the need for additional testing. CT provides adequate visualization of many causes of abdominal pain including an abdominal aortic aneurysm, diverticulitis, pancreatitis, appendicitis, and obstruction. It is better than a plain film of the abdomen to see free air. Spiral CT scan is comparable to an intravenous pyelogram (IVP) to evaluate stones. Ultrasound is best for biliary pathology. An MRI is useful for some things including pancreatic cancer, but often is not better than a CT scan. A colonoscopy should not be done in the setting of acute diverticulitis or perforation.

91. The answer is a. (*South-Paul, pp 348–368.*) The patient describes the classic presentation for peptic ulcer disease. Infection with *Helicobacter pylori* is the leading cause of peptic ulcer disease, with the use of NSAIDs the second most common cause. Alcoholism and gallstones can cause pancreatitis, but that presents differently. Gastroparesis may cause dyspepsia, but is a less likely cause for ulcer disease.

92. The answer is a. (*South-Paul, pp 348–368.*) Reflux can be appropriately diagnosed by medical history and by evaluating the response to treatment. Those who respond are likely to have the diagnosis. Upper endoscopy fails to reveal GERD in 24–50% of the patients who have been found to have GERD by a pH probe. EGD should be performed if bleeding, weight loss, or dysphagia is present, especially in an elderly patient. The other tests have not been shown to be sensitive or specific enough to replace response to treatment as a diagnostic tool.

93. The answer is d. (*South-Paul, pp 348–368.*) ERCP is the gold standard for diagnosis and treatment of choledocholithiasis, and is usually performed in the setting of an acute cholecystitis with increased liver enzymes, amylase or lipase. Ultrasound shows stones, but is less sensitive for choledocholithiasis or for complications (abscess, perforation, and pancreatitis). CT or MRI is better for those. HIDA can be used, and a negative one rules out cholecystitis, but in the setting of increased liver enzymes, an ERCP is a better choice.

94. The answer is a. (*South-Paul, pp 348–368.*) Gallstones cause about 50% of cases of pancreatitis. Alcohol causes about 30%. Ten to thirty percent are idiopathic. Less common causes include iatrogenic (for instance, after an ERCP), or hyperlipidemia.

95. The answer is c. (*South-Paul, pp 348–368.*) Amylase is sensitive, but not specific. Lipase is also sensitive, but more specific, as virtually all lipase is pancreatic in origin. If it is more than three times normal, it is very sensitive and specific. White blood cell count, glucose, and transaminases can be elevated, but are better used to assess prognosis, not make the diagnosis.

96. The answer is b. (*South-Paul, pp 348–368.*) Ranson's criteria assess the severity and prognosis of pancreatitis. On admission, 5 criteria are considered. It is a poor prognostic sign if the age is more than 55, white blood cell is greater than 16,000, glucose is greater than 200, LDH is greater than 350, and AST is greater than 250. Six other criteria reflect the development of complications and include a decrease in hematocrit greater than 10 mg/dL, a BUN increase greater than 5 mg/dL, calcium less than 8 mg/dL, PaO_2 less than 60 mmHg, base deficit greater than 4 mEq/L and a fluid sequestration greater than 6 L. These are assessed during the first 48 hours of admission.

97. The answer is b. (*South-Paul, pp 348–368.*) The Rome consensus committee for irritable bowel syndrome developed diagnostic criteria for IBS. These criteria include:

- Symptoms for at least 12 weeks (not necessarily consecutive) in 12 months
- Characterized by two of the following symptoms:
  - Relief with defecation
  - Onset associated with a change in stool frequency
  - Onset associated with a change in stool appearance

Crohn's disease and ulcerative colitis are inflammatory bowel diseases. Ulcerative colitis is likely to have perirectal pain with bloody diarrhea. Crohn's disease is likely to have right lower quadrant pain with weight loss. Lactose intolerance and diverticulitis are less likely to present this way.

98. The answer is d. (*Penner, Majumdar*) The patient is presenting with symptoms consistent with obstruction. In this case, abdominal radiographs are crucial in the decision making process, and to rule in/rule out a surgical abdomen. A fecalith is a hard stony mass of feces that can obstruct the appendix or a diverticuli. Without a fever or other evidence of appendicitis, that would be a less likely finding. In a perforation, x-ray would show free intraperitoneal air, but this patient's presentation is more consistent with obstruction. Stool may be seen on an abdominal film, but constipation would not likely present with the symptoms listed above. Gallstones are less likely to be seen on plain film.

99. The answer is d. (*Mengel, pp 9–12.*) Many types of cervical and vaginal abnormalities can be detected using the Pap smear. When the results are reported as "atypical squamous cells of undetermined significance" (ASCUS), the physician may repeat the test in 4–6 months and in 1 year, perform HPV testing on the sample, or proceed to colposcopy. If the HPV testing is negative, the patient is at low risk for cancer, and the Pap test can be repeated in 1 year, especially if the patient is monogamous.

100. The answer is d. (*Mengel, pp 9–12.*) When the results of a Pap smear are reported as ASCUS, and HPV testing on the sample is positive, the physician should proceed to colposcopy. Colposcopy involves cervical examination under stereoscopic magnification and includes biopsy of abnormal appearing areas, and is the definitive test for assessing Pap smear abnormalities. Imiquimod (Aldara) is an immune modulator and can treat warts, but is not indicated in this case.

101. The answer is c. (*Mengel, pp 9–12.*) When the results of a Pap smear are reported as ASCUS, and HPV testing is unavailable, the physician may choose to perform colposcopy or repeat the Pap smear in 4–6 months. If the physician chooses to repeat the Pap smear, the results should be carefully followed. If the results are reported as ASCUS or higher, a colposcopy should be performed. If the repeat is normal, the Pap should be repeated again in 4–6 months. If the repeat Pap smear is again negative, the frequency of testing can return to normal.

102. The answer is d. (*Mengel, pp 9–12.*) When the results of a Pap smear are reported as ASCUS, favoring low-grade intraepithelial lesion (LSIL), the physician should proceed to colposcopy. Colposcopy involves cervical examination under stereoscopic magnification and includes biopsy of abnormal appearing areas, and is the definitive test for assessing Pap smear abnormalities. If the biopsies confirm the diagnosis, definitive treatment is needed.

103. The answer is d. (*Mengel, pp 9–12.*) When the results of a Pap smear are reported as "atypical glandular cells," the physician should proceed to colposcopy. Colposcopy involves endocervical sampling, and will help to further identify the glandular cell abnormality noted on the Pap smear.

104. The answer is e. (*Mengel, pp 9–12.*) When the results of a Pap smear are reported as AGC, and are reported to be of endometrial origin, endometrial biopsy is necessary to rule out endometrial cancer. This is true even if the patient does not report abnormal vaginal bleeding.

105. The answer is b. (*South-Paul, pp 369–382.*) Iron deficiency may be asymptomatic, but patients may present with varying degrees of weakness, fatigue, dizziness, palpitations, or exercise intolerance. On physical examination, one may see pallor and tachycardia. Pica, the craving of ice, clay, or other unnatural substances is particularly associated with iron deficiency. Lead, anemia of chronic disease, B-12 and folate deficiency usually does not cause pica.

106. The answer is b. (*South-Paul, pp 369–382.*) Oral iron therapy is available as iron salts. One 300 mg tablet of iron sulfate delivers 60 mg of elemental iron. One 300 mg tablet of iron gluconate only delivers 34 mg of elemental iron. Absorption of iron is improved in an acidic environment, thus tablets are often given with ascorbic acid to improve absorption. For the same reason, antacids should be avoided with iron. Other things that inhibit iron absorption are calcium, soy proteins, and tannins (often found in tea and wine).

107. The answer is a. (*South-Paul, pp 369–382.*) The laboratory evaluation in this patient clearly indicates iron deficiency anemia. The most common cause is blood loss. Poor nutrition and/or inadequate absorption are less common causes. Chronic disease would lead to a high or normal ferritin and a low TIBC. Folic acid deficiency would lead to an elevated MCV.

108. The answer is e. (*South-Paul, pp 369–382.*) The laboratory results indicate anemia of chronic illness, in this case type 2 diabetes. It is likely a result of trapping of iron stores in the reticuloendothelial system, mild decrease in erythropoietin production and decreased marrow response to erythropoietin. Although elevated iron and erythropoietin may help slightly, the mainstay of his treatment is treating the underlying condition. Transfusions may be necessary preoperatively if the hemoglobin is less than 10 mg/dL.

109. The answer is d. (*South-Paul, pp 369–382.*) The patient described has a laboratory profile suspicious for thalassemia minor. These patients have low hemoglobin and MCV, but in contrast to iron deficiency, the patients have an elevated RBC and normal RDW. Additionally, the MCV is low out of proportion to the anemia. Given that the patient is asymptomatic, he should be treated only if necessary. Treatment includes transfusion if blood loss leads to significant anemia. The patient should have genetic counseling if planning a family.

110. The answer is c. (*South-Paul, pp 369–382.*) Some clinical features are common to all megaloblastic anemias—anemia, pallor, weight loss, fatigue, and glossitis to name a few. Neurological symptoms are specific to vitamin B-12 deficiency. Usually, treatment is parenteral vitamin B-12 replacement weekly for 1 month, often with concurrent administration of folic acid. Once levels are established, oral therapy may be sufficient.

111. The answer is e. (*South-Paul, pp 369–382.*) Most often, vitamin B-12 deficiency is a result of inadequate absorption. Since B-12 is present in all animal products, only strict vegans or people not ingesting animal products would be deficient from a dietary standpoint. Vitamin B-12 deficiency is not a side effect of hydrochlorothiazide. Alcohol can impact intracellular processing of folic acid, but not vitamin B-12.

112. The answer is b. (*South-Paul, pp 369–382.*) The slide shows sickle cell anemia, an autosomal recessive trait seen in those of African, Mediterranean, or Asian heritage. It is found before age 6 in 90% of patients, with acute pain crises as the most common presentation. Prophylaxis for pain crises involves ensuring adequate oxygenation and hydration. Immunization against streptococcal infection is appropriate, as most patients are functionally asplenic. The patients often have daily prophylaxis with penicillin until the age of 5. Immunization and antibiotic prophylaxis does not, however, prevent pain crises. Chronic analgesics and scheduled transfusions have not been shown to reduce pain crises.

113. The answer is b. (*Mengel, pp 37–43.*) The skin lesions of Rocky Mountain spotted fever are typically red macules on peripheral extremities that become purpuric and confluent. Lyme disease typically presents as a slowly spreading anular lesion—erythema chronicum migrans. Tularemia is characterized by pain and ulceration at the bite site. Brown recluse spider bites most often present as local pain and itching, then a hemorrhagic bulla with surrounding erythema and induration. The black widow bite is a mild prick followed by pain at the bite site.

114. The answer is a. (*Mengel, pp 37–43.*) Lyme disease occurs in the New England states, New York, and Wisconsin, but can be seen sporadically in the West and Midwest. Rocky Mountain spotted fever occurs in the western mountain states, Tularemia in the west, brown recluse spider bites in the south central United States, and chiggers in the southern and midwestern United States.

115. The answer is c. (*Mengel, pp 37–43.*) This case describes the typical presentation and physical examination findings of head lice, including the typical erythematous popular rash and "nits" on the hair follicles. Fleas, bedbugs, scabies, and chiggers may all present with erythematous papules, but would have a different distribution and would not have associated nits.

116. The answer is d. (*Mengel, pp 37–43.*) This case describes the classic distribution of scabies. Sarcoptes scabiei burrow into intertriginous areas, wrists, or areas where clothing is tight next to the skin. The lesions of chigger bites are similar, but bites are typically found in a linear pattern over wrists, ankles, and legs. Bedbugs typically infest unclothed areas—the neck, hands, and face. Fleas typically bite the lower extremities, and lesions from body lice would not follow the pattern described.

117. The answer is c. (*Mengel, pp 37–43.*) After a cat bite, hospitalization is indicated only if the bite involves the tendon, joint capsule, bone, or hand. Bites from a domestic cat carry a small risk of rabies, and immune globulin is not indicated. If rabies is suspected, the cat can be observed or tested. Treatment for the person can begin up to 8 days after exposure. Cat bites can become infected with pasturella multocida, which is sensitive to amoxicillin/clavulanate, but not clindamycin. Subcutaneous sutures are not recommended when closing a bite wound, as they are more likely to become infected.

118. The answer is b. *(Castells)* Typical local reactions to stings include swelling, erythema, and pain at and around the site of the sting. In general, they resolve quickly and minimal analgesia is all that is necessary. Large local reactions include extended areas of swelling that last several days. They are not allergic in origin, and carry a minimal risk of anaphylaxis upon reexposure. Toxic systemic reactions are associated with nausea, vomiting, headache, vertigo, syncope, convulsions, and fever. Pruritis, erythema and urticaria are less common. Persons who have a toxic reaction are at risk for anaphylaxis with subsequent stings. The reaction described in the above question is not anaphylactic in nature.

119. The answer is a. *(Mengel, pp 44–48.)* Gynecomastia is a benign enlargement of the male breast. It may be asymptomatic or painful, bilateral or unilateral. It commonly occurs around the time of puberty, and if so, requires only a history, physical examination, and reassurance if there are no abnormalities found. Most cases resolve within 1 year. Outside of the pubertal period, assessment of hepatic, renal, and thyroid functions may help uncover a cause. Sex hormones are only tested if progressive enlargement is noted.

120. The answer is c. *(Mengel, pp 44–48.)* Fibrocystic changes are the most common benign condition of the breast. Cysts may range in size from 1 mm to more than 1 cm in size. Fibroadenomas are usually rubbery, smooth, well-circumscribed, nontender, and freely mobile. Mammograms are not necessary for women under 30, as they are less sensitive in younger women with denser breast tissue. Mastitis generally occurs with nursing, and is characterized by inflammation, edema, and erythema in areas of the breast.

121. The answer is d. *(Mengel, pp 44–48.)* Up to 15% of breast cancers are mammographically silent. Therefore, a palpable mass deserves further workup, even if the mammogram is negative. Workup may include an ultrasound to determine if the mass is cystic or solid, and possible biopsy. Aspiration of the mass may be appropriate, but biopsy is still necessary if the mass is palpable after aspiration, if the fluid is bloody, or if the mass reappears within 1 month. The characteristics of the fluid otherwise does not dictate workup. Genetic testing is of no value in the workup of a breast mass, but can be considered based on family history, and under the direction of an experienced genetic counselor.

122. The answer is e. (*Mengel, pp 44–48.*) Patients with mastitis should be encouraged to continue nursing, and should be started on an antibiotic that covers streptococcus and staphylococcal infections. Reducing caffeine and methylxanthines, or using evening primrose oil may decrease symptoms of fibrocystic breast disease, but has no impact on mastitis. Applying heat may help symptoms, but ice will not have the desired effect.

123. The answer is a. (*Mengel, pp 44–48.*) Spontaneous, unilateral discharge is most suspicious for breast cancer. The characteristics of the discharge cannot be used to distinguish benign versus malignant causes, however, bloody, serous, serosanguineous, or watery discharge deserve a workup.

124. The answer is c. The degree of abnormality seen on a mammogram is classified using the breast imaging reporting and date system (BI-RADS) system. BI-RADS classification 0 means that the test was incomplete, and additional testing should be conducted as soon as possible. BI-RADS 1 and 2 mean that the mammogram is benign, and routine screening can be conducted at usual intervals. BI-RADS 3 indicates that the lesion is probably benign, but that diagnostic mammogram should be performed in 6 months. BI-RADS 4 and 5 are suspicious for, and highly suggestive of, cancer (respectively) and that tissue diagnosis is needed.

125. The answer is d. (*Mengel, pp 48–54.*) Hand cellulitis often follows puncture wounds, and cat bites may often produce infection with *P. multocida*. Most skin infections are due to *S. aureus or S. pyogenes. C. perfringens* may produce gas, and should be considered as a cause for cellulitis that can lead to gangrene, especially if creptius is found on clinical examination. *H. influenzae* sometimes infects the skin of younger children.

126. The answer is c. (*Mengel, pp 48–54.*) Hot tub folliculitis is commonly seen in the setting described in this question. Often, the infection is self-limited, but occasionally antibiotics with pseudomonal coverage are necessary. While streptococcal and staphylococcal species are common causes of folliculitis, in the case of recent hot tub use, Pseudomonas is more likely. Tinea and candida do not generally cause folliculitis.

127. The answer is b. (*Mengel, pp 48–54.*) The child in this case has the classic presentation of impetigo. Most cases of impetigo are caused by either streptococcal or staphylococcal skin infections. When staphyloccus is the infecting organism, the lesions are generally bullous with minimal erythema. When streptococcus is the infecting organism, there is erythema with a typical golden crust that occurs after the lesion ruptures. While impetigo often occurs in the setting of an acute viral infection, the skin infection is not a result of the virus itself. Pneumococcus and haemophilus may cause skin infections, but typically not impetigo.

128. The answer is c. (*Mengel, pp 48–54.*) Acne is a potentially chronic skin condition that can have severe physical and social consequences. Classification of acne is the prime determinant of management and is based on the severity and type of lesions present. Comedonal acne involves impaction of the pilosebaceous follicle. Open comoedones (blackheads) and closed comedones (whiteheads) generally respond best to topical retinoids. These agents are comedolytic. Inflammatory acne is characterized by pustules and surrounding erythema, and generally responds best to antibiotic therapy (topical if more mild, oral if more severe) either alone or in combination with topical retinoids or benzoyl peroxide. Severe nodular or cystic acne may require oral isoretinoin.

129. The answer is a. (*Goldstein*) Tinea infections are common, and may be spread by close person-to-person contact (as in school wrestling). The classic tinea lesion is pruritic, erythematous, with raised borders, and central scaling. This can often be confused with eczema or a bacterial skin infection, but by scraping the lesion and visualizing hyphae with microscopic examination, the diagnosis of tinea can be confirmed. Tinea cruris occurs in the groin, not on the thigh, Pityriasis rosea has a different classic appearance.

130. The answer is a. (*Meisel*) When someone presents to the office complaining of chest pain, the history is invaluable in helping determine if the pain is due to a life-threatening cause (myocardial infarction, pulmonary embolism, aortic dissection or tension pneumothorax, to name a few). Studies have shown that the likelihood of myocardial infarction with a chest pain history increases when pain is said to:

- Radiate to the right, left, or both arms/shoulders
- Be exertional
- Be associated with diaphoresis
- Be associated with nausea or vomiting

- Be described as a "pressure"
- Be described as worse than previous cases of angina, or similar to past MI

The likelihood decreases when the pain is described as pleuritic.

131. The answer is c. (*Meisel*) Historical features are important when determining likely causes of chest pain. In the case described, several of the symptoms are nonspecific, and may be related to any of several etiologies. Shortness of breath is possible in asthma, PE, ischemia, or bronchitis. Cough is also possible in asthma, PE, and bronchitis. Pain that is worse with lying down is more commonly associated with a PE, but the key feature here is the abrupt onset. In general, musculoskeletal pain not associated with trauma has a vague onset. Pain from asthma and bronchitis is usually not abrupt. Pain from myocardial ischemia is usually gradual as well, and associated with activity.

132. The answer is c. (*Meisel*) Nitroglycerine may relieve the pain of myocardial ischemia, but is not reliable enough to distinguish between ischemia and other noncardiac causes of chest pain. Relief of pain with a GI cocktail is similarly unreliable. If pain is relieved with eating, it is likely GI in origin, and if it is relieved with sitting up and leaning forward, pericarditis is likely. Relief with activity cessation is strongly suggestive of ischemic pain.

133. The answer is a. (*Light*) Given his history and physical examination findings, the patient is likely to have a spontaneous pneumothorax. Of the options listed, chest tube insertion may be the most appropriate therapeutic intervention. Antibiotics, bronchodilators, anticoagulation, and aspirin may be appropriate with other diagnoses, but not in this case.

134. The answer is e. (*Meisel*) Hypertension is a risk factor for coronary artery disease and aortic dissection. "Heartburn" is not a feature suggestive of myocardial ischemia. A recent viral infection may precede an episode of pericarditis or myocarditis. His smoking history is certainly significant, but not as important as his history of drug use. His physical examination findings (diaphoresis and agitation) are more consistent with a stimulant use, likely cocaine. The risk of myocardial infarction increases 24 times that of baseline in the 60 minutes after cocaine use.

135. The answer is d. (*Mengel, pp 54–60.*) Pain that is increased with palpation is most often associated with a musculoskeletal etiology. In this case, treatment with NSAIDs is most appropriate. A chest x-ray and bloodwork is not necessary at this time. An ECG might be indicated if there were risk factors for coronary artery disease, but based on this patient's symptoms and lack of concerning historical features, it would not be necessary. A proton pump inhibitor would not be indicated for pain that is worsened with palpation.

136. The answer is e. (*Mengel, pp 54–60.*) The ECG shown has no acute changes, but is suggestive of left ventricular hypertrophy. Her symptoms are quite suggestive of angina. Since she is currently asymptomatic and her ECG shows nothing acute, transfer to the hospital is unwarranted. The best approach would include patient education for warning signs, and some sort of stress testing. For women in her age group, stress ECGs are often falsely positive, so a stress test with imaging is most appropriate.

137. The answer is d. (*Meisel*) Syncope associated with chest pain may be seen with aortic dissection. Hemodynamic instability may be associated with a PE, a ruptured aortic aneurysm or critical aortic stenosis. The physical examination findings described, including the murmur and carotid pulse findings (pulsus parvus et tardus), are very suggestive of aortic stenosis.

138. The answer is a. (*Meisel*) Exercise ECG testing is simple and inexpensive. It is not useful in the face of an abnormal resting ECG (ST segment changes, left ventricular hypertrophy, Wolff Parkinson White syndrome or paced rhythm). Chemical stress tests or tests with imaging are reserved for those who cannot exercise or those who have baseline ECG abnormalities. Catheterization would not be indicated, and Electron beam CT scanning is not clinically useful in this setting.

139. The answer is d. (*Meisel*) According to the 2002 ACA/AHA guidelines, beta blockers should be discontinued for four to five half-lives (typically around 48 hours) prior to stress testing if possible. The drug should be withdrawn gradually. Hydrochlorothiazide does not interfere with stress testing.

140. The answer is d. (*Mengel, pp 72–81.*) The differential diagnosis for an acute cough includes asthma exacerbation, acute bronchitis, aspiration, exposure to irritants (cigarette smoke, pollutants), allergic rhinitis, uncomplicated pneumonia, sinusitis with postnasal drip, and viral upper respiratory infection. Of these usual causes, viral upper respiratory infection is by far the most common cause. Viral URIs is the most frequent illness in humans with a prevalence of up to 35%.

141. The answer is a. (*Mengel, pp 72–81.*) The most common causes of a chronic cough are asthma, postnasal drainage, smoking, and gastroesophageal reflux disease. Given that he did not respond to a bronchodilator, asthma is an unlikely diagnosis. Pertussis would have likely responded to azithromycin, and is therefore not likely to be the correct answer in this case. His associated symptoms of sore throat and sour taste in his mouth, combined with symptoms that are worse when lying down make GERD the most likely diagnosis. Medication side effects should be considered, with the ACE inhibitors most likely to cause a cough.

142. The answer is b. (*Mengel, pp 72–81.*) Because the patient reports a productive cough for at least 3 months of the year for at least 2 consecutive years, she meets the criteria for chronic bronchitis. This is the most common cause of chronic cough in smokers. While it is true that her smoking may cause irritation of her airways, it wouldn't explain why the cough isn't present year-round (since she continues to smoke throughout the year). The most common cause of chronic cough in nonsmokers is postnasal drainage, but since this patient has a significant smoking history, chronic bronchitis is more likely. Lung cancers rarely present solely with cough. Associated signs and symptoms include weight loss and hemoptysis. Asthma is less likely to present with a productive cough.

143. The answer is e. (*Mengel, pp 72–81.*) The Centers for Disease Control published guidelines for treating acute bronchitis. The guidelines state the antibiotics are not indicated for uncomplicated acute bronchitis, regardless of the duration of the cough. Antibiotics should be reserved for patients with significant chronic obstructive pulmonary disease (COPD), CHF, those who are very ill appearing or the elderly. This patient likely has hyper-responsive airways, sometimes called a post-bronchitic cough. In this case, the best treatment would be an inhaled steroid or oral steroid taper. Anti-inflammatory medications and nasal steroids are not effective.

144. The answer is d. (*Mengel, pp 72–81.*) Antibiotics do not alter the course of pertussis unless initiated early in the illness. However, antibiotics do prevent transmission and decrease the need for respiratory isolation from 4 weeks to 1 week, and are therefore recommended. The first-line antibiotic choice is either erythromycin for 14 days, or azithromycin for 5 days. Amoxicillin and amoxicillin/clavulanate are not effective.

145. The answer is a. *(Mengel, pp 95–104.)* Acute diarrhea is defined as an increased number or decreased consistency of stool lasting 14 days or less. Most acute diarrhea is due to infection and usually occurs after the ingestion of contaminated food or water, or direct person-to-person contact. Viral infections account for 70–80% of acute infectious diarrhea, with Rotavirus being the most frequent cause. Enteric adenoviruses are the second most common type. Rotavirus occurs in the winter months, and most cases occur between the ages of 3 months and 2 years. Contaminated water, salads, or shellfish may transmit Norwalk virus. Giardiasis is less common in the general population, but may be more prevalent in children in daycare centers. *Salmonella* is generally due to raw or undercooked meat, and enterotoxigenic *E. coli* is the most common cause of traveler's diarrhea.

146. The answer is e. *(Mengel, pp 95–104.)* Approximately one-third of travelers to underdeveloped countries will develop travelers' diarrhea. Of those, 40% will alter their plans because of the symptoms, 20% will be bed-bound for at least 1 day, and 1% will require hospitalization. Most cases of travelers' diarrhea are due to enterotoxigenic *E. coli*. The other causes of diarrhea are less likely in this setting.

147. The answer is b. *(Mengel, pp 95–104.)* The antibiotic of choice for travelers' diarrhea is a flurorquinolone (ciprofloxacin, ofloxacin, or norfloxacin) with trimethoprim/sulfamethoxazole or azithromycin being acceptable alternatives. The other antibiotics listed may be useful for other causes of diarrhea, but are not indicated for travelers' diarrhea.

148. The answer is c. *(Mengel, pp 95–104.)* IBS is a complex of abnormal GI motility, altered visceral sensation and psychological factors that occurs in about 20% of the U.S. population. Most of those affected develop symptoms before age 35, and women are twice as likely as men to suffer from symptoms. The Manning criteria help to differentiate IBS from organic pathology. Four or more criteria make the diagnosis likely, and presence of less than two make the diagnosis less likely. The criteria include pain relief with bowel movement, more frequent bowel movements with the onset of pain, looser stools with the onset of pain, passage of mucus, sensation of incomplete evacuation, and abdominal distension. Giardiasis would generally cause more watery diarrhea, *E. histolytica* would generally cause daily symptoms with bloody diarrhea and malaise, inflammatory bowel disease would generally present with bloody diarrhea and weight loss, and lactose intolerance would generally be associated with ingestion of lactose.

149. The answer is e. (*Mengel, pp 95–104.*) For acute viral diarrhea, adults should be encouraged to eat potatoes, rice, wheat, noodles, crackers, bananas, yogurt, boiled vegetables, and soup. Dairy products, alcohol, and caffeine should be avoided. Oral rehydrating solutions can be used if vomiting is a problem, and fasting is not indicated. Avoidance of wheat, barley, and rye is indicated for celiac disease, but not for acute viral diarrhea.

150. The answer is d. (*Mengel, pp 105–108.*) "Dizziness" is a subjective symptom, often meaning different things to different people. It is imperative that this complaint be better characterized to develop an appropriate differential diagnosis and treatment plan. Vertigo is a rotational sensation, in which the room spins around the patient. Orthostasis refers to a lightheadedness upon arising, common with orthostatic hypotension. Presyncope is a feeling of impending faint. Disequilibrium is a sensation of unsteadiness, or a loss of balance. If asked whether the problem is in the head or the feet, patients often respond by saying the problem is in the feet. Lightheadedness is often vaguely described as a "floating" sensation.

151. The answer is c. (*Mengel, pp 105–108.*) Acoustic neuroma typically presents with unilateral tinnitus and hearing loss. The symptoms are constant and slowly progressive. With continued tumor growth, symptoms of vertigo, facial weakness, and ataxia occur. Vestibular neuronitis presents with an acute onset of severe vertigo lasting several days, with symptoms improving over several weeks. Benign positional vertigo typically involves symptoms with position changes only. Meniere's disease presents with discreet attacks of vertigo lasting for several hours, associated with nausea and vomiting, hearing loss, and tinnitus. A cerebellar tumor would typically present with dysequilibrium as opposed to tinnitus.

152. The answer is a. (*Mengel, pp 105–108.*) The Dix-Hallpike maneuver, described in the question, is often useful to distinguish central from peripheral causes of vertigo. With a peripheral cause of vertigo, the latency time for the onset of symptoms of vertigo or nystagmus is 3–10 seconds, the symptoms are severe, and the direction of the nystagmus is fixed. In addition, repeating the maneuver lessens the symptoms. With a central cause of vertigo, there is no latency to onset of symptoms, no lessening of symptoms with repeat maneuvers, the direction of the nystagmus changes, and the symptoms are of mild intensity. Of the above answers, all are peripheral causes of vertigo, except the correct answer, stroke.

153. The answer is b. *(Mengel, pp 105–108.)* Once diagnosed with a peripheral vestibular disorder, antihistamines are the first-line therapy for symptomatic relief. They suppress the vestibular end organ receptors and inhibit activation of the vagal response. Meclizine (Antivert), 25 mg orally every 4–6 hours and diphenhydramine (Benadryl), 50 mg orally every 4–6 hours are commonly recommended choices. Antiemetics may be used if nausea and vomiting are prominent symptoms. Benzodiazepines may be helpful in symptom reduction, but are usually second-line agents. NSAIDs and antibiotics are not helpful.

154. The answer is a. Brain imaging is indicated in the workup of dizziness if history and examination cannot reliably distinguish between central or peripheral causes. MRI and magnetic resonance angiography (MRA) are the tests of choice, although a CT scan cutting through the cerebellum may be an alternative if MRI isn't available. Audiometry is used to distinguish between cochlear versus retrocochlear causes of peripheral vertigo. Brainstem evoked audiometry is used to detect acoustic neuromas, and electronystagmography does not distinguish between central and peripheral problems.

Barton J, Branch WT. Approach to the patient with vertigo. http://www.utdol.com/utd/content/topic.do?topicKey=genneuro/2118&type=A&selectedTitle=2~29. Accessed 8/21/2006.

155. The answer is e. *(Mengel, pp 116–121.)* Those at risk for obstructive lung disease include pediatric patients (asthma, bronchitis, bronchiolitis), adults with asthma and adults with chronic cigarette smoking. Dyspnea due to restrictive lung disease is more likely with occupational exposures (for farmers, cotton dust, grain dust, and hay mold), those with severe scoliosis, the morbidly obese and pregnant patients.

156. The answer is b. *(Mengel, pp 116–121.)* Gullain-Barre syndrome causes dyspnea due to respiratory muscle paralysis or dysfunction. A main clinical feature is bilateral symmetric progressive weakness. Parkinson's disease and ALS generally present in an older population. Lyme disease can cause a polyneuropathy, but is unlikely without other symptoms. Psychogenic weakness and dyspnea is less likely with these clinical findings.

157. The answer is c. *(Mengel, pp 116–121.)* Symptoms of pneumonia include dyspnea, cough, sputum production, and occasionally pleuritic chest pain. Signs include fever, tachypnea, rales, dullness to percussion, and egophony. Asthma, PE, and CHF would be less likely to be associated with a fever, and bronchitis would be unlikely to be associated with egophony.

158. The answer is e. (*Mengel, pp 116–121.*) The patient is presenting with signs and symptoms of CHF. These include abnormal heart sounds (a murmur or an additional heart sound), cardiomegaly, JVD, basilar rales, and dependent edema. Bronchodilators would be appropriate for asthma or bronchitis. Antibiotics may be appropriate for pneumonia. Steroids would be helpful with an asthma or COPD exacerbation. Anticoagulation may be appropriate for a deep venous thrombus.

159. The answer is b. (*Mengel, pp 116–121.*) Asthma in children is characterized by recurrent episodes of wheezing. Bronchiolitis and pneumonia may also cause wheezing, but would be less likely to be recurrent. Congenital heart disease can also cause dyspnea and even cyanosis with exertion, but are less likely to cause wheezing.

160. The answer is d. (*Mengel, pp 116–121.*) The signs and symptoms in this case indicate a deep venous thrombus causing a PE, likely due to oral contraceptives. The treatment of choice would be anticoagulation.

161. The answer is a. (*Mengel, pp 116–121.*) B-type natriuretic peptide evaluates for the presence of CHF. Studies indicate that a value less than 80 pg/mL has a high (99%) negative predicative value and helps rule out CHF.

162. The answer is e. (*Mengel, pp 116–121.*) A d-dimer test is useful in determining the risk for a DVT or PE. A low result has a high negative predictive value for the presence of thrombus. If the result were high, a confirmatory test would be appropriate. A spiral CT scan has become a standard validated test. A V/Q scan, often used in the past, can be used when a spiral CT is unavailable, but is often indeterminate. A pulmonary angiogram is the gold standard. Doppler flow studies are used to verify a DVT. If positive, a PE can be assumed in the correct clinical setting.

163. The answer is d. (*Mengel, pp 116–121.*) Many studies have shown that opioids relieve dyspnea in patients with cancer, but the mechanism is unknown. Bronchodilators are better in the setting of COPD and asthma, as are steroids. Anxiolytics help, but seem to relieve the anxiety associated with dyspnea more than the dyspnea itself. Pulmonary rehabilitation would be an inappropriate step in a dying patient.

164. The answer is a. (*Mengel, pp 121–126.*) A recent meta-analysis found that four factors correlate significantly with a diagnosis of acute bacterial cystitis. They are frequency, hematuria, dysuria, and back pain. In addition, four factors decrease the likelihood of UTI (absent dysuria, absent back pain, history of vaginal discharge, and history of vaginal irritation). Women with any combination of the positive and negative symptoms have a more than 90% probability of a UTI. Urethritis is more likely with a gradual onset. Patients with pyelonephritis often have fever. Interstitial cystitis tends to be more chronic in nature, and is generally not associated with back pain. Vulvovaginitis is a common cause of dysuria, but is associated with vaginal irritation or discharge.

165. The answer is a. (*Mengel, pp 121–126.*) Urine culture is indicated when acute bacterial cystitis is suspected, but the urinalysis leaves the diagnosis in question. Therefore, in the setting of classic symptoms but a negative dipstick or microscopic evaluation, a culture will confirm the diagnosis. In the other cases, either the urine dipstick or microscopic evaluation confirms the clinical suspicion, and culture is not indicated.

166. The answer is d. (*Mengel, pp 121–126.*) In 85% of women with recurrent UTIs, symptoms develop within 24 hours of sexual intercourse. If measures like voiding after intercourse, acidification of the urine and discontinuing diaphragm do not work, prophylaxis is indicated for women with frequent infections. Single-dose postcoital antibiotic use is often helpful. If that does not decrease infections, daily single dose antibiotic prophylaxis may be appropriate for 3–6 months. If symptoms reoccur after discontinuation of daily prophylaxis, it may need to continue for 1–2 years.

167. The answer is b. (*Mengel, pp 121–126.*) Dysuria without pyuria is common. In the postmenopausal years, atrophy is a usual cause. In younger women, a careful history can reveal a bladder irritant (caffeine and acidic foods are common irritants). When hematuria is present, interstitial cystitis should be suspected. Interstitial cystitis is generally diagnosed through cystoscopy, based on the presence of ulcerations and fissures in the bladder mucosa and the absence of bladder tumors. Urodynamic studies often demonstrate a small bladder capacity, with urge to void with as little as 150 mL of fluid in the bladder.

168. The answer is b. (*Mengel, pp 121–126.*) The American College of Obstetrics and Gynecology recommends treating asymptomatic bacteriuria in pregnancy, as 20–35% of the cases eventually develop into overt UTIs. In the other cases above, treatment of asymptomatic bacteriuria is not indicated, as it has not been shown to decrease morbidity and may increase the likelihood of developing resistant microorganisms.

169. The answer is e. (*Mengel, pp 376–383.*) In men with urinary symptoms and a normal urinary tract, UTIs are not the norm, and cystitis and pyelonephritis are uncommon causes. Urethritis would be unlikely to cause this systemic illness. The patient described above has acute bacterial prostatitis. Acute prostatitis is most commonly seen in 30- to 50-year-old men, and symptoms include frequency, urgency, and back pain. The patient appears acutely ill, and has pyuria. The prostate examination would reveal a boggy, tender, and warm prostate.

170. The answer is a. (*Mengel, pp 126–132.*) The peak age range for the diagnosis of acute otitis media is 6 months to 7 years. Native Americans and Eskimos experience acute otitis media more frequently than do people of other races. Children with cleft palate or Down syndrome are also at increased risk. Children in group daycare, and children whose parents smoke are also at increased risk. Children with heart murmurs have not been shown to be at increased risk, and parental history of allergies has not been shown to be a direct risk factor.

171. The answer is e. (*Mengel, pp 126–132.*) Hearing impairment is common with acute otitis media and eustacean tube dysfunction. It can also be associated with barotrauma, and may be coupled with tinnitus and vertigo. It may occur with otitis externa, if the ear canal is so edematous that it is nearly occluded, or if discharge is occluding the canal. Hearing loss would be unlikely in temporomandibular joint syndrome.

172. The answer is b. (*Mengel, pp 126–132.*) The patient has temporomandibular joint dysfunction, a common cause of referred otalgia. The first line of therapy includes treatment with NSAIDs, heat, a mechanical soft diet, and referral to the dentist if there is no improvement in 3–4 weeks. Antibiotic therapy is not indicated. Obtaining an MRI would not add value to the diagnosis or treatment plan at this stage. An erythrocyte sedimentation rate may be elevated in temporal arteritis, another cause of referred ear pain, but would not be likely to be useful in this setting.

173. The answer is d. *(Mengel, pp 126–132. South-Paul, pp 41–65.)* A reddened tympanic membrane, by itself, is not a sufficient finding to diagnose acute otitis media. It may be due to increased intravascular pressure associated with crying. More reliable findings include an opaque tympanic membrane (indicating a purulent effusion), a bulging tympanic membrane and impaired tympanic membrane mobility. When all three of those characteristics are present, the positive predictive value is near 90%. Purulent discharge in the ear canal may indicate a tympanic membrane perforation, and in the face of an otherwise normal canal is more indicative of acute otitis media than otitis externa.

174. The answer is a. *(Mengel, pp 126–132.)* Effusions may take up to 3 months to resolve. Antibiotics are not indicated for persistent effusions in the absence of acute otitis media. Effusions persisting beyond 3 months require evaluation by an otolaryngologist. Decongestants or antihistamines have never been documented to help effusions, but may be symptomatically helpful.

175. The answer is b. *(South-Paul, pp 41–65.)* Although there are many risk factors for otitis media, the primary one is daycare. Participation in group daycare substantially increases the number of pathogens to which a child is exposed. Less important risk factors include an increased number of siblings in the home, exposure to cigarette smoke, pacifier use, formula use, and lower socioeconomic status. Children with cleft palate or Down syndrome are at a greatly increased risk. Family history has not been identified as a risk factor, and vaccines have not been shown to decrease the incidence of otitis media. Because otitis media is often caused by nontypeable *H. influenzae* and by strains of pneumococcus not covered by the pediatric 7-valent vaccine, up to date immunizations have not proven to decrease the risk for otitis media.

176. The answer is d. *(Mengel, pp 126–132.)* The patient described has temporomandibular joint syndrome, a common cause of ear pain. Antibiotics are of no use. NSAIDs with a mechanical soft diet are the first line therapy of choice. If this is not helpful, referral to a dentist may be appropriate for a bite guard is appropriate. Physical therapy would not be helpful as a first line therapy, but may be necessary if a bite guard isn't helpful.

177. The answer is b. *(Mengel, pp 126–132.)* The picture represents acute otitis media. The child should be treated with a first-line antibiotic, and of those listed, amoxicillin is the best choice. Azithromycin is often used as a first-line choice in 1-day, 3-day, or 5-day doses, but it should be reserved as a second-line therapy.

178. The answer is a. (*Taylor, pp 600–606.*) Since *S. pneumoniae* is the leading bacterial cause of otitis media, it was hoped that the introduction of the pneumococcal vaccine would significantly decrease the occurrence of otitis. However, the vaccine has been associated with about a 6% reduction in the number of episodes of acute otitis media, and about a 10% reduction in the frequency of recurrent acute otitis. Although this decline is not as dramatic as hoped, the vaccination would prevent up to 1.2 million episodes of acute otitis in the United States each year.

179. The answer is b. (*Taylor, pp 600–606.*) The first-line treatment for otitis externa ("swimmer's ear") is topical antibiotics. Systemic antibiotics are rarely indicated, unless there is an acute otitis media associated with it, or when there is local spread of the infection. Flushing the ear canal is not indicated, and may be harmful unless the tympanic membrane can be visualized and is without perforation. Topical hydrocortisone can be added to the antibiotic, and may help resolve symptoms, but is not effective treatment by itself. Oral steroids are not indicated.

180. The answer is c. (*Mengel, pp 132–136.*) There are many medications known to cause peripheral edema as a side effect. Antihypertensives such as calcium channel blockers are well-known to cause this, but direct vasodilators, beta blockers, centrally acting agents and antisympathetics also can cause edema. Of the diabetic medications, insulin sensitizers such as rosiglitazone often cause edema. Hormones, corticosteroids, and nonsteroidal anti-inflammatory agents also cause problems. SSRIs like fluoxetine do not commonly cause this symptom. Neither does ACE inhibitors like lisinopril or thiazide diuretics.

181. The answer is b. (*Mengel, pp 132–136.*) The leg swelling due to lipedema is due to an abnormal accumulation of fatty substances in the subcutaneous tissues and is commonly mistaken for lymphedema. The condition spares the feet, distinguishing it from lymphedema. Hepatocellular disease and venous insufficiency would cause edema and would be unlikely to spare the feet. Varicose veins will often cause edema, but once again would be unlikely to spare the feet.

182. The answer is e. *(Mengel, pp 132–136.)* In the workup of edema, the first thing to note is if the edema is bilateral or unilateral. Bilateral edema associated with signs and symptoms of CHF (dyspnea, rales, or JVD) would necessitate a chest x-ray to rule in the diagnosis, followed by an echocardiogram. If ascites is present, liver function studies are needed. If these are absent, the clinician should check an urinaysis. If the sediment is abnormal, nephritic syndrome or acute tubular necrosis (ATN) is the likely diagnosis.

183. The answer is c. *(Mengel, pp 132–136.)* In the workup of edema, the first thing to note is if the edema is bilateral or unilateral. Bilateral edema associated with dyspnea, rales, or JVD would necessitate an evaluation for CHF. If ascites is present, liver function studies are needed.

184. The answer is d. *(Mengel, pp 132–136.)* In the workup of edema, the first thing to note is if the edema is bilateral or unilateral. Unilateral edema not associated with trauma or signs of infection requires a Doppler ultrasound to evaluate for the presence of DVT.

185. The answer is e. *(Mengel, pp 132–136.)* Unilateral edema is suspicious for a DVT. However, if there is a history of recent trauma, or evidence of inflammation, a Doppler ultrasound is usually not necessary. Signs of inflammation including erythema point toward cellulitis as a diagnosis.

186. The answer is c. *(Mengel, pp 132–136.)* In patients with chronic venous insufficiency, knee-length elastic stockings can aid venous return. Additional treatment options include leg elevation throughout the day. Prolonged standing should be limited. Unilateral edema usually does not respond to diuresis, sodium restriction, or an ACE inhibitor. The case described above would be unlikely to be related to a DVT because of its chronic nature.

187. The answer is c. *(Mengel, pp 137–140.)* It is important to classify enuresis correctly, as treatment may vary depending on type. Enuresis is classified as primary if it has never followed a period of dryness. Enuresis that occurs after 6 months of dryness is classified as secondary enuresis. Enuresis is nocturnal if it only happens at night, and diurnal if it happens during the day and at night. There is no classification of "primary intentional enuresis."

188. The answer is a. *(Mengel, pp 137–140.)* While the cause of nocturnal enuresis is unknown, it is felt to be due to decreased production of nocturnal antidiuretic hormone. It is not likely due to deep sleep, though most enuretic patients do not spontaneously awaken after bedwetting. It is associated with a maturational delay, and statistically 25% of 5-year-olds are enuritic. The numbers decrease about 15% per year. Forty to fifty percent of bedwetters are female. Family history is very important. If one parent was enuretic, there is a 40% likelihood that the child will be. If both parents were bedwetters, there is a 70% risk that the child will be. Interestingly, the child will usually stop around the same time that the parent did. Very few patients have an organic cause.

189. The answer is b. (*Mengel, pp 137–140.*) Enuresis alarms have been shown to be the most effective treatment for nocturnal enuresis. Initial cure rates are high, and relapse rates are low. The alarms need to be used appropriately, with parental involvement in order to be effective. Frequent nighttime wakening may be effective, but compliance is a barrier to effectiveness. DDAVP can also be effective, but relapse rate is high once the medication is discontinued. Tricyclics have a lower initial cure rate and a high relapse rate. They can also be lethal, if overdosed. Oxybutynin has a high relapse rate and has not been proven to be efficacious when compared with placebo.

190. The answer is a. (*Rakel, pp 838–840.*) In the child with monosymptomatic nocturnal enuresis, no further evaluation is needed, other than a thorough voiding history, physical examination, and urinalysis. X-rays of the lumbar and sacral spine are indicated if there is suspicion of spina bifida occulta, and renal ultrasound/VCUG are indicated if there are suspected anatomic abnormalities that would lead to enuresis.

191. The answer is a. (*Rakel, pp 838–840.*) Treatment for nocturnal enuresis should be first directed at treating constipation. It often coexists, and when constipation is treated, the situation improves dramatically. Motivational therapy should be considered for families not interested in pharmacologic therapy, but should never include consequences for wetting. The child has no control over wet nights, and should never be punished for a wet bed. DDAVP, a synthetic analog of vasopressin, works well in the form of a nasal spray or oral pill, but should not be the first measure tried. Imipramine is a tricyclic antidepressant with anticholenergic side effects, including urinary retention. It is useful, but not as an initial measure. Tolterodine is a treatment for overactive bladder, and has not been shown to be helpful for simple nocturnal enuresis.

192. The answer is a. *(Rakel, pp 838–840.)* Moisture-sensitive alarms can be a very successful behavioral treatment for nocturnal enuresis. The first drops of urine complete a circuit, activating an alarm that will wake the child (and the parents). The parents then help the child complete voiding in the toilet. Over time, a conditioned response develops, and the child awakens voluntarily with the sensation of a full bladder. There is no gender difference in success rates, and with appropriate use and parent involvement, success rates are between 70% and 90%. It may take weeks or months to be successful, and requires a sizeable commitment from the parents and child involved. The child should not take responsibility for this treatment, because without parental involvement, success rates drop.

193. The answer is a. *(South-Paul, pp 16–24.)* The growth chart raises concern for failure to thrive. In the United States, the vast majority of failure to thrive is secondary to inadequate nutrition and a thorough dietary history is most likely to reveal the cause. Albumin has a long half-life, and is a poor indicator of recent undernutrition. Prealbumin is decreased in acute inflammation and undernutrition, and is therefore insensitive. Organic disease, including hypothyroidism, is found in less than 10% of cases of failure to thrive. IgA levels are sensitive to undernutrition and would be decreased in failure to thrive.

194. The answer is d. *(South-Paul, pp 16–24.)* In a child with failure to thrive diarrhea and recurrent respiratory infections, cystic fibrosis must be considered, and a sweat chloride test should be ordered. The other tests may be indicated in the workup of failure to thrive, but only with a reasonable degree of clinical suspicion. With the history given, the most useful test would be the sweat chloride test.

195. The answer is a. *(South-Paul, pp 16–24.)* Familial short stature has a growth curve that shows simultaneous changes in height and weight. In failure to thrive and constitutional growth delay, weight decreases first, then height. In hypothyroidism, height velocity slows first and may plateau before weight changes. In breast-fed infants, weight decreases relative to peers after 4–6 months, but catches up after 12 months.

196. The answer is e. *(South-Paul, pp 16–24.)* Hospital admission is indicated for failure to thrive, in the face of hypotension and bradycardia. Other interventions may be appropriate, but with vital sign abnormalities, it is important to admit the patient. Patients like this are generally not neglected, especially since he has been seen all along for well child checks.

197. The answer is d. (*Wolff, pp 548–550.*) Mononucleosis is often mistaken for streptococcal pharyngitis. Both have symptoms of sore throat, fatigue, fever, and adenopathy. If patients with mononucleosis are given ampicillin (and other penicillin derivatives), they often develop the rash described above, sometimes confused as an allergic reaction to penicillin. The rash of scarlet fever is more confluent, and has a sandpaper-like texture.

198. The answer is c. (*Mengel, pp 147–152. Taylor, pp 465–469.*) The most common causes of fatigue in primary care include depression, life stress, chronic medical conditions, and medication reactions. Red flags for other causes include all of the symptoms listed in this question. Chronic fatigue syndrome can be associated with unrefreshing sleep, postexertional fatigue, difficulty with concentration, and headaches. It is usually not associated with weight loss, and if that sign is present, one should look for other causes for fatigue.

199. The answer is a. (*Mengel, pp 147–152.*) Depression is one of the most common diagnoses in patients presenting with fatigue, especially when denying weakness or hypersomnolence. Once the complaint is defined, the practitioner should screen for depression. Screening for sleep apnea, anemia, hypothyroidism, and pregnancy should happen if the screen is negative.

200. The answer is b. (*Mengel, pp 147–152.*) There are three general categories of fatigue: Physiologic, physical, and psychological. Physiologic fatigue is generally due to overwork, lack of sleep, or a defined physical stress, such as pregnancy. Physical fatigue is due to infections, endocrine imbalances, anemia, cardiovascular diseases, and more concerning causes like cancer. Psychological fatigue is generally associated with stress, depression, anxiety, or adjustment reaction. While all types of fatigue can last for 6 months, the progressive nature of this patient's symptoms should lead one to look for a physical cause. Increased stress, overwork, and alcohol use generally do not point to a physical cause of stress.

201. The answer is d. (*Mengel, pp 147–152.*) The initial laboratory workup for an uncertain diagnosis of fatigue included a complete blood count, sedimentation rate, urinalysis, chemistry panel, thyroid testing, pregnancy test (for women of childbearing age), and age/gender appropriate cancer screening. In a 55-year-old African American male, a prostate screen would be appropriate. Chest x-ray, ECG, HIV test, and a drug screen would be appropriate if the initial screen is negative.

202. The answer is e. *(Mengel, pp 174–178.)* Meckel's diverticulum is the most common cause of significant GI bleeding in children. It is a congenital abnormality that occurs in about 2% of the population, with a male to female ration of 2:1. It occurs about 2 feet from the ileocecal valve, and is usually about 2 in long. About 2% of cases have complications. These facts are often remembered as "the rule of 2s." Intussusception also occurs in this age group, but is usually painful. Anal fissures, colitis, and juvenile polyposis generally do not cause significant bleeding.

203. The answer is c. *(Mengel, pp 174–178.)* Upper endoscopy is the best diagnostic testing option in the setting of an acute upper GI bleed. It can localize the source of bleeding, potentially allow therapeutic intervention, and allow for tissue diagnosis when necessary. Gastric lavage is less useful, and a barium study might interfere with subsequent intervention. Red cell scans are better to locate bleeding sources in the lower GI tract, and angiography may miss slower bleeds.

204. The answer is d. *(Rakel, pp 617–621.)* Meckel's diverticulum is the most common congenital abnormality of the GI tract, present in about 2% of the population. Most are asymptomatic, but a common presentation is painless large-volume intestinal hemorrhage. A Meckel's diverticulum is often incidentally diagnosed at laparotomy. A noninvasive diagnostic modality is the technetium scan, often called the "Meckel's scan." The labeled tracer is picked up by the heterotopic gastric mucosa in the diverticulum. A Meckel's diverticulum is located in the distal ileum, and would not be identified by the other endoscopic procedures above.

205. The answer is c. *(Rakel, pp 617–621.)* Approximately 5–15% of patients with colonic diverticulosis develop severe diverticular bleeding. While many believe it may be triggered by the ingestion of indigestible foods, that has never been proven by studies. It is unusual to find the source of bleeding using colonoscopy. If colonoscopy does not localize the bleeding, a tagged red blood cell scan should be the next step, and will help guide segmental resection if necessary. A subtotal colectomy is only necessary for recurrent severe bleeding with no source identified.

206. The answer is e. *(Rakel, pp 639–643.)* The condition described is a thrombosed external hemorrhoid. External hemorrhoids are defined as hemorrhoids arising distal to the dentate line. When they thrombose, they are associated with acute pain and are hard and nodular on physical examination. The treatment can be safely done in the office with local anesthesia. It eliminates pain immediately and eliminates the risk of reoccurrence. Hydrocortisone would not be helpful. Rubber band ligation and sclerotherapy should be reserved for internal hemorrhoids. Incision and drainage of the hemorrhoid increases the risk of reoccurrence and can lead to infection of the retained clot.

207. The answer is a. *(Rakel, pp 639–643.)* An anal fissure is a split in the anoderm of the anal canal. It generally occurs after the passage of a hard bowel movement. Patients present with excruciating pain on defecation with blood found on the toilet paper. After the bowel movement, the patient may complain of an ache or spasm that resolves after a couple of hours. Thrombosed external hemorrhoids would generally be visible on examination. Internal hemorrhoids are generally not painful, unless they are thrombosed because of an unreducible prolapse. If that were the case, the pain would not resolve. A peri-anal abscess may not present with bleeding, but would likely be associated with systemic signs of infection.

208. The answer is c. *(Taylor, pp 528–536.)* In patients with headaches, the history is the most important way to characterize the headache. Migraine headaches are usually unilateral, but so are cluster headaches. Unilateral symptoms are less helpful in differentiating between the two. Nausea is associated with migraine, and is less likely to be associated with cluster or tension headaches. Rhinorrhea and sweating are symptoms more commonly seen with cluster headaches.

209. The answer is a. *(Taylor, pp 528–536.)* While any and all of the choices listed as answers may be necessary in the initial evaluation of a headache, the most important way to characterize the headache is by history. Physical examination would be confirmatory. Blood work, imaging, and consultation may be important in the management, but only after the characterization of the headache as migraine, cluster, tension, or secondary headache.

210. The answer is a. *(Taylor, pp 528–536.)* While many agents have been used as prophylactic agents to prevent migraines, beta-blockers are the most studied, and are effective. Verapamil is the only calcium channel blocker that studies show to have a prophylactic effect. There has been some interest in fluoxetine for prophylactic therapy, but more studies are needed. Ergotamines are used for abortive therapy.

211. The answer is b. *(Taylor, pp 528–536.)* Of the choices listed, tricyclic antidepressants are the only agents proven to have additive effects in migraine prophylaxis.

212. The answer is e. *(Taylor, pp 528–536.)* Narcotics have almost no place in migraine therapy. In well-controlled studies, the use of antiemetic injections or injectable ergotamines is more likely to be helpful, and is superior to narcotics. If acetaminophen or NSAIDS are ineffective, it usually means the dose is subtherapeutic, or there is a failure to absorb the medication because of vomiting or gastric stasis.

213. The answer is b. *(Taylor, pp 528–536.)* Verapamil appears to have some migraine prophylactic effect, but there is no evidence that other calcium channel blockers have a similar effect. Other calcium channel blockers may be helpful in suppressing cluster headaches, but have not been shown to be helpful for migraines.

214. The answer is d. *(Taylor, pp 528–536.)* The mainstay of therapy for cluster headaches is to provide relief from the acute attacks, then use therapy to suppress headaches during the symptomatic period. Nifedipine has been shown to be effective, as has prednisone, indomethacin and lithium. However, the medication should not be given daily, just during the symptomatic period. Fluoxetine has not been shown to be beneficial, and ergotamine is generally only helpful in the acute stage—not for prophylaxis.

215. The answer is e. *(Taylor, pp 528–536.)* Cluster headaches characteristically develop rapidly, achieving peak intensity within 10–15 minutes. Usually, the headaches are intensely painful and last for about 2 hours without treatment. The mainstay of treatment is oxygen, but many patients do not have access to this in their homes. In general, oral medications do not act rapidly enough to provide relief to the patients in the acute phase. Therefore, injectable or inhaled medications are preferred. Inhaled ergotamine has been shown to be helpful, as has injectable sumatriptan. Interestingly, local anesthetics administered into the nostril on the affected side have also been shown to be effective.

216. The answer is b. (*Taylor, pp 528–536.*) Tension-stress (or muscle contraction) headaches have a formal definition, with positive and negative criteria for diagnosis, but many physicians diagnose this type of headache by exclusion (after ruling out more interesting or rare etiologies for headache). They are in fact, the most frequent of all headaches encountered in clinical practice. The episodes last from 30 minutes to several days, and headaches should occur less than 15 times per month. It requires at least two of the following characteristics:

- Pressure/tightness
- Bilateral
- Mild to moderate
- Not aggravated by activity

There is generally no nausea. Either photophobia or phonophobia may be present, but not both. If criteria for this classification of headache are met, a trial of NSAIDs may be appropriate, with follow up if no improvement. Narcotics should be avoided, since the condition is generally chronic, and overuse is likely. Imaging would not be helpful or indicated at this stage.

217. The answer is e. (*Taylor, pp 528–536.*) A common question in family medicine relates to whether or not to obtain radiological imaging in the case of headache. In general, these characteristics should raise suspicion, and imaging should be considered:

- Headaches of recent onset or those that seem to become steadily more severe
- Headaches that do not fit any of the primary classifications
- Headaches that do not respond to first-line treatment
- Headaches associated with development of neurological abnormalities

218. The answer is b. (*Mengel, pp 219–223.*) There are several medications that can cause hematuria. They include penicillins, cephalosporins, sulfonamides, phenytoin, cyclophosphamide, mitotane, anticoagulants, and nitrofurantoin. Ibuprofen may cause kidney problems, but hematuria is not one of them. Oral contraceptives, SSRIs and diuretics do not commonly cause hematuria.

219. The answer is a. (*Mengel, pp 219–223.*) Cystitis is associated with suprapubic pain, dysuria, urgency, and frequency. In women, it is a very common diagnosis, and can usually be treated based on symptoms and the result of a urinalysis only. Pyelonephritis is generally associated with systemic signs of infection. Nephrolithiasis would cause hematuria, but would not be associated with dysuria or frequency. Bladder cancer is usually asymptomatic, but does cause hematuria. A sexually transmitted infection generally does not cause hematuria, but can cause dysuria and frequency.

220. The answer is e. *(Mengel, pp 219–223.)* Painless hematuria without other symptoms is the most common presentation of bladder carcinoma. Risk factors include being male, smoking and working in the printing/leather dye insustries. Acute prostatitis and a UTI are usually associated with dysuria, fever, and urinary frequency and urgency. Chronic prostatitis is associated with urinary symptoms as well. Stones are associated with pain.

221. The answer is d. *(Mengel, pp 219–223.)* Pseudohematuria can be derived from chemical agents, foods, or vaginal bleeding. Common foods that cause this include beets, blackberries, and rhubarb. Medications that discolor the urine include chloroquine, metronidazole, phenytoin, rifampin, and sulfasalazine, among others.

222. The answer is a. *(Mengel, pp 219–223.)* Terminal hematuria suggests either a bladder neck or a prostatic urethral lesion. Hematuria occurring throughout micturition occurs with bladder or renal lesions. Urolithiasis is associated with pain, and although urethral trauma is associated with hematuria, it would occur throughout micturition.

223. The answer is e. *(Mengel, pp 219–223.)* In a pediatric patient with hematuria, red cell casts and an elevated creatinine, glomerulonephritis is possible. Poststreptococcal infection accounts for 50% of all cases of pediatric hematuria. The other tests described above would identify stones or tumors, but those are unlikely in this age group.

224. The answer is a. *(Mengel, pp 219–223.)* In patients under forty with hematuria, but a normal IVP and urine culture, periodic monitoring and reassurance is appropriate. In a patient more than 40, cystoscopy or renal biopsy would be appropriate. A poststreptococcal glomerulonephritis would be unlikely in this age group, and a renal biopsy would not be needed if the creatinine is normal.

225. The answer is c. *(Rakel, pp 648–655.)* Hepatitis A is the most commonly reported hepatitis virus, and does not lead to chronic infection. Fecal shedding of the virus occurs early, and is no longer an issue at the time of presentation. Infectiousness is highest during the prodrome, and actually decreases by the time jaundice develops. Relapses of hepatitis A are rare, but do occur. Fulminant liver disease occurs in less than 1% of patients.

226. The answer is b. *(Rakel, pp 648–655.)* Hepatitis B infection is clearly associated with an increased risk of developing hepatocellular carcinoma, and has been labeled as having oncogenic properties.

227. The answer is a. *(Rakel, pp 648–655.)* Transmission of Hepatitis B may occur through the transfer of blood or body fluids, but can also occur perinatally (vertical transmission). If the virus is acquired early in life, the infection is silent, but up to 90% of those infected develop chronic disease. Those with a compromised immune system may also develop chronic disease easier than healthy patients. Healthy adults infected have spontaneous resolution more than 95% of the time. As with infection with hepatitis A, a small percentage of those infected will develop fulminant liver disease.

228. The answer is a. *(Rakel, pp 648–655.)* Identifying the correct stage of Hepatitis B infection relies heavily on the correct interpretation of serologic markers. The first marker to appear after infection is usually Hepatitis B surface antigen. It may appear prior to the onset of clinical symptoms, and usually disappears in a few weeks as the patient recovers. Hepatitis B core antigen is a protein contained in the inner core of the virion and is not found in the serum. The antibody to the core protein is found early, and persists indefinitely. The hepatitis B e antigen correlates with active replication.

229. The answer is a. *(Rakel, pp 648–655.)* Unlike HBV, the hepatitis C virus has not been found in body fluids other than blood, and the virus is primarily transmitted through exposure to blood and blood products.

230. The answer is c. *(Rakel, pp 648–655.)* The HBsAG positivity in this case indicates either chronic infection or early infection. The negativity of the IgM anti-HBc rules out an early infection. The HBeAg is correlated with replication, as is the HBV DNA.

231. The answer is e. *(Rakel, pp 648–655.)* The positivity of the anti-HBs indicates either exposure with immunity, recovery phase, or vaccination. Because the IgG anti-HBc is negative, there is no evidence of past exposure or infection.

232. The answer is a. *(Rakel, pp 648–655.)* The HBsAG positivity in this case indicates either chronic infection or early infection. The positivity of the IgM anti-HBc indicates early infection, and is negative in chronic infection. If the patient were in the recovery phase, his HBsAg would be negative.

233. The answer is b. *(South-Paul, pp 506–517.)* Contrary to common perception, urinary incontinence is not inevitable with aging. However, many common age-related changes do predispose elderly patients to incontinence. It is important to remember that these changes are found in many healthy, continent elderly persons. Involuntary bladder contractions increase with age. Total bladder contractility decreases with age. Elderly patients excrete a larger percentage of fluid late in the day (increasing nocturia), and urogenital atrophy leads to decreased internal urethral sphincter sensitivity.

234. The answer is d. *(South-Paul, pp 506–517.)* Asymptomatic bacteriuria is common in well elderly, and does not cause incontinence—whereas, a symptomatic infection may. Hyperglycemia can cause secondary incontinence because of polyuria, and continence can be restored by more tightly controlling the pateint's sugar. Diuretics also may cause secondary incontinence, and may need to be avoided unless necessary. Stool impaction is thought to be a causative factor in up to 10% of patients with incontinence, and disimpaction may restore continence. Atrophic vaginitis may also be causative, and treatment may improve the situation.

235. The answer is c. *(South-Paul, pp 506–517.)* Urge incontinence is the most common type of incontinence in the elderly. Due to detrusor hyperactivity, patients often complain of a strong urge followed by an involuntary loss of urine. Functional incontinence refers to a limitation that does not allow the patient to void in the bathroom (bed rest, paralysis, severe dementia) and does not generally relate to the urinary tract. Stress incontinence is the loss of urine associated with increased abdominal pressure, and overflow incontinence is incontinence due to overdistention of the bladder. Senile incontinence is a fictional term.

236. The answer is d. *(South-Paul, pp 506–517.)* Stress incontinence is much more commonly seen in women than in men, and is most often caused by urethral hypermobility resulting from weakness of the pelvic floor musculature. Patients complain of involuntary loss of urine associated with increases in intra-abdominal pressure (when sneezing, coughing, laughing, or exercising). Functional incontinence refers to a limitation that does not allow the patient to void in the bathroom (bed rest, paralysis, severe dementia) and does not generally relate to the urinary tract. Urge incontinence is the loss of urine following a strong urge, and overflow incontinence is incontinence due to overdistention of the bladder. Senile incontinence is a fictional term.

237. The answer is e. (*South-Paul, pp 506–517.*) Overflow incontinence is primarily a loss of the ability to empty the bladder, usually due to neurogenic bladder (longstanding diabetes, alcoholism, disk disease) or because of outlet obstruction (prostatic enlargement). Incontinence is usually a frequent or constant leakage of small amount, but occasionally a large amount of urine is lost without warning. Functional incontinence refers to a limitation that does not allow the patient to void in the bathroom (bed rest, paralysis, severe dementia) and does not generally relate to the urinary tract. Stress incontinence is the loss of urine associated with increased abdominal pressure, and urge incontinence is preceded by a strong urge to urinate. Senile incontinence is a fictional term.

238. The answer is e. (*South-Paul, pp 506–517.*) After ruling out secondary causes of incontinence, a postvoid residual measurement should be taken. This can be done through catheterization or via ultrasound. A postvoid residual less than 50 mL is normal. A postvoid residual greater than 200 mL indicates inadequate bladder emptying and is consistent with overflow incontinence. Between 50 and 200 mL is indeterminate.

239. The answer is b. (*South-Paul, pp 506–517.*) Kegel exercises are designed to strengthen the pelvic floor musculature. Patients are asked to squeeze the muscles in the genital area as if they were trying to stop the flow of urine from the urethra. They hold this contraction for 10 seconds, and repeat this many times in the day. Patients are then taught to contract these muscles and hold them during situations where incontinence may occur. They are most useful to treat stress incontinence, but may help with mixed incontinence as well. It is not helpful for functional, urge, or overflow incontinence.

240. The answer is a. (*South-Paul, pp 506–517.*) Pharmacological therapy is indicated for incontinence if a behavioral approach is ineffective. For urge incontinence, anticholinergic medications are the drugs of choice with oxybutynin (Ditropan) and tolterodine (Detrol) both indicated for symptoms. Pseudoephedrine has been shown to help stress incontinence, trimethoprim-sulfamethoxazole has been shown to help in the case of prostatitis, and finasteride and terazosin will help frequent voiding caused by prostatic hyperplasia.

241. The answer is a. (*South-Paul, pp 170–184.*) Primary amenorrhea is defined as the absence of menses at age 16 in the presence of normal secondary sex characteristics, or absence of menses at age 14 in the absence of secondary sex characteristics. It is usually the result of a genetic or anatomic abnormality. Gonadal dysgenesis is the most common cause of primary amenorrhea, responsible for about 50% of the cases. The most well-known type is Turner's syndrome (45 XO). Hypothalamic failure is often a result of anorexia nervosa, excessive exercise, chronic or systemic illness and severe stress, and results from a suppression of hypothalamic GnRH secretion. Pituitary failure may result from inadequate GnRH stimulation and is often associated with a history of head trauma, shock, infiltrative processes, pituitary adenoma, or craniopharyngioma. These patients will often display deficiency of other pituitary hormones as well. PCOS may cause primary amenorrhea, but is generally associated with normal breast development. Constitutional delay of puberty, although common in boys, is an uncommon cause of amenorrhea in girls, but clinically is very hard to distinguish from other more common causes.

242. The answer is c. (*South-Paul, pp 170–184.*) Pregnancy is the most common cause of secondary amenorrhea, and can even occur in a patient who claims that she has not been sexually active or says that she only has intercourse during "safe" times. Polycyctic ovarian syndrome is common, and is responsible for about 30% of the cases of secondary amenorrhea. It is characterized by androgen excess, and symptoms include irregular or absent menses, hirsuitism, acne, and virilization. Functional hypothalamic amenorrhea is usually a result of anorexia, rapid weight loss, rigorous exercise, or significant emotional stress. Hypothyroidism and hyperprolactinemia can both be associated with secondary amenorrhea, but are less common causes.

243. The answer is c. (*South-Paul, pp 170–184. Mengel, pp 387–391.*) Anovulatory bleeding is caused by continuous unopposed endometrial estrogen stimulation. Since these patients do not ovulate, progesterone from the corpus luteum is not secreted, the withdrawal from which would normally cause endometrial sloughing. It is the most common cause of dysfunctional uterine bleeding in women younger than 20 years of age, accounting for about 95% of cases. When women are within 2 years of menarche, this is especially common, and can be followed expectantly. Alternatively, oral contraceptives can be used to regulate periods. Pregnancy should be ruled out, even in women who deny sexual activity. Ovulatory bleeding due to fluctuations in estrogen and progesterone levels is also a cause of abnormal bleeding, but accounts for only about 10% of cases. Leiomyomas and polyps may cause bleeding, but usually not in this age group.

244. The answer is d. (*Mengel, pp 387–391.*) If a postmenopausal woman has vaginal bleeding, she needs an endometrial biopsy to rule out endometrial cancer. In fact, this is usually the first step in the evaluation of this problem, after performing the examination and ruling out sexually transmitted infections or anatomic abnormalities. Ultrasound evaluation may be needed, but this would not be the next step in the evaluation of this condition. Contraindications to this procedure include pregnancy, acute infection, PID, or known bleeding disorder (including coumadin use).

245. The answer is a. (*South-Paul, pp 170–184.*) Primary dysmenorrhea is caused by the release of prostaglandin from the endometrium at the time of menstruation. Treatment focuses on the reduction of endometrial prostaglandin production. This can occur either by using medications that inhibit prostaglandin synthesis, or by suppressing ovulation. NSAIDs are generally the first line of therapy, given their favorable risk/benefit ratio and effectiveness. They should be started the day before menstruation, if possible. Daily use of NSAIDs does not increase effectiveness, and is associated with an increase of side effects. While opiate use may help with pain control, it does not inhibit prostaglandin synthesis and may lead to addiction. SSRI therapy is sometimes used for premenstrual dysphoric disorder, but is not a first-line therapy for dysmenorrhea. OCPs can be used and are effective, but are thought of as second-line therapy.

246. The answer is a. (*Mengel, pp 13–17.*) Turner's syndrome is the most common karyotypic abnormality associated with amenorrhea. It is associated with short stature, a webbed neck, and sexual infantilism.

247. The answer is b. (*Mengel, pp 13–17.*) Many medications can cause hyperprolactinemia leading to amenorrhea. When hyperprolactinemia is related to medication, the measured prolactin level is usually less than 100 ng/mL. Many psychotropic medications can cause this, including benzodiazepines, SSRIs, tricyclic antidepressants, phenothiazines, and buspirone. Neurologic drugs that can increase prolactin levels include sumatriptan, valproate, and ergot derivatives. Estrogens and contraceptives can also elevate prolactin, as can some cardiovascular drugs (atenolol, verapamil, reserpine, and methyldopa). This is a less likely side effect in proton pump inhibitors, diuretics, ACE inhibitors, and thyroid replacement.

248. The answer is e. (*Mengel, pp 13–17.*) The progestin challenge test separates patients with estrogen deficiency from those with normal or excess estrogen. Any bleeding in the week after the administration of Provera indicates that the patient has sufficient estrogen to menstruate, and that the amenorrhea is likely due to anovulation. Those with premature ovarian failure would not have a withdrawal bleed. Neoplasm, Turner's syndrome and Asherman's syndrome would not likely present in this way.

249. The answer is a. (*Mengel, pp 13–17.*) Patients with amenorrhea and elevated testosterone and DHEA-S levels need CT scanning of the adrenal glands and ultrasound of the ovaries to rule out neoplasm.

250. The answer is a. (*Mengel, pp 13–17.*) When evaluating primary amenorrhea in patients with normal secondary sexual characteristics and a normal initial laboratory evaluation (pregnancy test, thyroid stimulating hormone, and prolactin level), it is appropriate to perform a progestin challenge test. When there is no withdrawal bleeding, it either indicates inadequate estrogen production or an outflow tract obstruction. An estrogen-progestin challenge can differentiate between the two. No withdrawal bleeding after an estrogen-progestin challenge indicates an outflow tract obstruction or an anatomic defect.

251. The answer is a. (*Mengel, pp 13–17.*) Primary dysmenorrhea is defined as pain with menstruation, not associated with identified pelvic pathology. Secondary dysmenorrhea is associated with identified pelvic pathology. In general, if the history and physical examination are normal, no further workup is necessary, and a trial of treatment is indicated. Gonorrhea and Chlamydia cultures may be necessary in the initial evaluation, but if the history and examination are not suggestive of infection, cultures are not necessary. Ultrasound, hysterosalpingography, and laparoscopy are not indicated at this stage of the evaluation.

252. The answer is a. (*Mengel, pp 108–112.*) The history above is classic for primary dysmenorrhea (not associated with pelvic pathology). Pain from endometriosis usually begins several days before menses and may last throughout the entire cycle. Leiomyomas (fibroid tumors) are generally asymptomatic. When symptoms are present, it is usually described as pelvic pressure, bloating menorrhagia or metorrhagia, depending on the tumor size or location. Adenomyosis is usually associated with severe pain and menorrhagia. The pain associated with ovarian cysts is different than that described.

253. The answer is b. (*Mengel, pp 13–17.*) OCPs suppress menstrual fluid volume and prostaglandin release. This is done by causing endometrial hypoplasia.

254. The answer is a. (*Mengel, pp 60–66.*) Delirium and dementia are often clinically difficult to distinguish, especially if you are unfamiliar with the patient. Disorientation is characteristic of both processes, as is a disturbed sleep-wake cycle. His history of hypertension would lead one to think of multi-infarct dementia, rather than delirium. Responsiveness to questions may be a feature of either process, though patients with delirium often have a shortened attention span. The abrupt onset of a mental status change is consistent with delirium as opposed to dementia, which occurs insidiously.

255. The answer is c. (*Mengel, pp 60–66.*) The patient described has a hypertensive encephalopathy. With his severe hypertension, a stroke may be considered, but unlikely without focal neurological deficits. Sixth nerve palsy may be seen in a stroke. Pinpoint pupils would be more consistent with narcotic excess, unlikely given his vital signs and history. Dilated pupils suggests sympathetic outflow, and may be consistent with delirium tremens, but the history and physical is not consistent with this. Papilledema is seen with hypertensive encephalopathy. Anisocoria of 1 mm is a nonspecific finding that can be seen in normal individuals.

256. The answer is d. (*Mengel, pp 60–66.*) Hyperalert confusion is common with alcohol withdrawal. Hypothyroidism would present with fatigue and psychomotor slowing. Fluoxetine usually does not cause a withdrawal syndrome, but may be associated with depressive symptoms. Opiate withdrawal does not present with a confusional state. Amphetamine withdrawal would be associated with psychomotor slowing.

257. The answer is e. (*Mengel, pp 60–66.*) While a urinalysis, complete blood count, toxicology screen, and pregnancy test may all reveal the cause of delirium, the patient's history is consistent with viral or bacterial meningitis. A lumbar puncture is the most likely test to reveal the diagnosis in this case.

258. The answer is c. *(Mengel, pp 60–66.)* In dementia, the level of consciousness is not clouded, but disorientation may occur later in the illness. Hypertension and diabetes may be seen with both delirium and dementia. The inability to complete serial sevens (count backwards from 100 by 7s) may be related to educational level. Although her symptoms have appeared recently, it is often difficult to pinpoint the exact onset of dementia. Delirium is seen as being more abrupt in onset.

259. The answer is c. *(Rakel, pp 5–10.)* While all of the medications listed above have antiemetic properties, the patient described has gastroparesis, likely as a result of her longstanding diabetes. Metoclopramide can improve gastric motility and help her symptoms more than the other antiemetics listed.

260. The answer is c. *(Rakel, pp 5–10.)* A careful history and physical examination can often distinguish between potential causes for nausea and vomiting. In this case, mild pain, followed by the acute onset of distension, nausea, and vomiting is consistent with ileus or obstruction. Hyperactive bowel sounds lead one to think of obstruction; with an ileus bowel sounds are absent. Gastroenteritis begins acutely, but is usually not preceded by mild abdominal pain. Diverticulosis and diverticulitis would cause pain, but would be less likely to present with nausea, vomiting, and distension.

261. The answer is b. *(Rakel, pp 5–10.)* Psychogenic vomiting should be suspected in patients who are able to maintain adequate nutrition despite chronic symptoms. It is usually seen during times of social stress or in patients with a past history of a psychiatric disorder. Chronic gastroenteritis is an unlikely condition. While young girls in this age group are at risk for anorexia and bulimia, sufferers usually do not seek medical attention or treatment until concerned others bring the condition to medical attention. A central nervous system malignancy is possible, if the lesion involves the vomiting center, but one would expect to see nutritional deficit in this case.

262. The answer is b. *(Rakel, pp 5–10.)* The situation described is consistent with viral gastroenteritis, a common clinical condition. The Norwalk virus, reoviruses, and adenoviruses are common causes. Symptoms typically begin acutely and are associated with typical viral syndrome symptoms. Generally, these illnesses are self-limited, and will resolve within 5 days. Oral rehydration is indicated as long as there are no signs of severe dehydration. Intravenous rehydration and antiemetics may have a role, but only in more severe cases. There is no role for antibiotic therapy.

263. The answer is d. (*Rakel, pp 5–10.*) The patient described has pancreatitis, likely due to gallstones. While the laboratory findings in acute pancreatitis are often nonspecific, elevated serum amylase in the right clinical setting is often suggestive. Radiographic evidence can help confirm the diagnosis. In establishing a cause for pancreatitis, history is key, but some laboratory findings are helpful. Elevated ALT is more suggestive of gallstone pancreatitis, and is less likely when alcohol or hypertriglyceridemia is the cause. ACE inhibitors are an uncommon cause of pancreatitis. Hypercalcemia is also a rare cause, but is unlikely in this case.

264. The answer is e. (*Mengel, pp 288–295.*) The symptoms and characteristics of nausea and vomiting can often be clues to the etiology. When nausea happens before eating in the morning, likely etiologies include pregnancy, uremia, alcohol withdrawal, and increased intracranial pressure (meningitis or space-occupying lesions). Gastroparesis and pancreatitis is usually associated with nausea after eating. Cholelithiasis is associated with nausea, vomiting, and pain after eating fatty foods. Vestibular disorders cause nausea without any clear association with meals or time of day.

265. The answer is a. (*Mengel, pp 288–295.*) Gastroparesis is associated with nausea and vomiting delayed 1 hour or more after eating. The vomit is nonbilious and the food is undigested. Nausea associated with cholelithiasis is associated with pain, usually after eating fatty foods. The nausea from pancreatitis is usually after meals, and is associated with pain. Vestibular disorders cause nausea without clear relationship to eating, and a brain tumor would cause morning symptoms.

266. The answer is c. (*Mengel, pp 288–295.*) Children with pyloric stenosis usually present with weight loss, dehydration, and occasionally a palpable "olive" mass in the epigastric area. It usually is identified before 7 weeks of age. Breast milk allergies are uncomomon. Reflux may be possible, but is less likely to be associated with weight loss and dehydration. Intussesception is associated with significant abdominal pain, and hemoccult positive stools. Small bowel obstructions are less likely, and are associated with high-pitched bowel sounds.

267. The answer is b. *(Mengel, pp 288–295.)* Pancreatitis is associated with the acute onset of significant nausea, vomiting, and epigastric pain. The symptoms occur after eating, and are improved when the patient does not eat. Amylase and lipase are likely to be abnormal, but the CBC is likely normal. Hemoccult testing, abdominal x-rays, and upper endoscopy are likely to be normal.

268. The answer is d. *(Mengel, pp 288–295.)* The patient described likely has cholelithiasis. Nausea, vomiting, and pain occur after eating fatty meals. The diagnostic test of choice would be a right upper quadrant ultrasound to identify stones in the gallbladder. Amylase and lipase may be positive if the patient develops secondary pancreatitis, but are unlikely to be elevated until that point. Hemoccult testing, abdominal x-rays, and upper endoscopy are all likely to be normal.

269. The answer is d. *(Mengel, pp 288–295.)* Antiemetics can cause a variety of side effects. The phenothiazines (Compazine and Phenergan) generally cause drowsiness, dry mouth, and dizziness. Tigan causes similar side effects. Zofran is a serotonin receptor antagonist, and may cause dizziness and headache. Reglan is a prokinetic agent, and can cause diarrhea and extrapyramidal reactions.

270. The answer is c. *(Mengel, pp 300–306.)* There are several characteristics of palpitations that can help the physician determine whether or not the symptoms are from a cardiac cause. These include male sex, the description of the symptom as an "irregular heartbeat," a personal history of heart disease, and event duration greater than 5 minutes. Family history of similar symptoms would not be a risk factor for cardiac disease.

271. The answer is a. *(Mengel, pp 300–306.)* When a patient describes her heartbeat as rapid and irregular, it suggests either atrial fibrillation or atrial flutter. Ectopy and atrial fibrillation can both cause an irregular pulse. PSVT is usually rapid and regular, as is stable ventricular tachycardia (VT). Stimulant abuse will generally cause a sinus tachycardia. While hyperthyroidism may cause atrial fibrillation, the patient would likely have other additional symptoms.

272. The answer is c. *(Mengel, pp 300–306.)* Ventricular premature beats are often random, episodic, and instantaneous beats, often described as a "flip-flopping" sensation. Atrial fibrillation is described more as a rapid and irregular heart rate or a "fluttering" in the chest. PSVT is generally rapid and regular, and lasting a longer time. Stimulant abuse would likely cause sinus tachycardia, and while hyperthyroidism can cause premature beats, the patient would likely experience other symptoms.

273. The answer is b. (Mengel, pp 300–306.) Hypertrophic cardiomyopathy can be associated with atrial fibrillation or ventricular tachycardia. The characteristic heart murmur associated with it is a systolic ejection murmur (like aortic stenosis) worsening with Valsalva's maneuver. Mitral valve prolapse would have a different characteristic murmur. Dilated cardiomyopathy and CHF would likely be associated with other symptoms. Atrial fibrillation would not be associated with a regular rhythm.

274. The answer is a. (Mengel, pp 300–306.) When the history, physical examination, 12-lead ECG and limited laboratory evaluation are negative, it is appropriate to reassure the patient with palpitations and continue observation. The likely etiology is benign supraventricular or ventricular ectopy. Other tests and consultation would only be indicated if the patient's symptoms are incapacitating or worrisome.

275. The answer is d. (Mengel, pp 300–306.) Since this patient's arrhythmia only seems to occur with exercise, stress testing would be useful. Ambulatory ECG monitoring and echocardiography would not be useful. Consultation with an electrophysiologist may be appropriate, depending on the results of the testing.

276. The answer is c. (Mengel, pp 300–306.) The classic WPW (preexcitation syndrome) ECG demonstrates a short PR interval and delta waves. Patients are treated if they have symptomatic arrhythmia. Treatment usually consists of radiofrequency ablation, but pharmacologic therapy is also an option.

277. The answer is c. (Mengel, pp 313–320.) Classically, ovarian cysts present with a unilateral dull pain that can become diffuse and severe if the cyst ruptures. On physical examination, the examiner feels a smooth mobile adnexal mass with peritoneal signs if the cyst ruptures. PID is associated with fever and vaginal discharge. Ectopic pregnancy may present with similar symptoms, but menses would not be normal. Uterine leiomyoma would be associated with an enlarged uterus, and appendicitis would be associated with nausea and anorexia.

278. The answer is a. (*Mengel, pp 313–320.*) Pelvic inflammatory disease is classically described as lower abdominal pain that is gradual in onset and bilateral. Fever, vaginal discharge, dysuria, and occasionally abnormal vaginal bleeding may be associated symptoms. The minimal diagnostic criteria include uterine, adnexal, or cervical motion tenderness. Treatment should provide coverage for likely etiologic agents (*N. gonorrhoeae, C. trachomatis,* anaerobes, and enteric gram-negative rods).

279. The answer is b. (*Mengel, pp 313–320.*) The pain associated with ectopic pregnancy is often described as colicky, and may radiate to the shoulder if there is a significant hemoperitoneum. Amenorrhea and symptoms of pregnancy are diagnostic clues.

280. The answer is e. (*Mengel, pp 313–320.*) The patient described has symptoms and signs suggestive of endometriosis. A complete blood cell count would be helpful if the signs are suggestive of an infectious process (appendicitis or PID). An erythrocyte sedimentation rate is elevated in 75% of patients with pelvic inflammatory disease, but is nonspecific. CA-125 levels may be helpful if the physician is concerned about an ovarian mass. Transvaginal ultrasound may be helpful, but MRI is more sensitive for localization of endometriosis.

281. The answer is c. (*Mengel, pp 313–320.*) Eighty percent of ovarian masses in girls younger than 15 years are malignant. Because of the high potential for malignancy, any adnexal mass should be evaluated by transvaginal ultrasound and referral for surgical removal. In many women of child-bearing years, adnexal masses are commonly cysts. If the pain is not acute or recurrent, palpable cysts less than 6 cm in size may be monitored with repeat pelvic examination. Ultrasound is reserved for those masses that do not resolve, or those that increase in size. CT and MRI may be useful in some cases, but the ultrasound is the best first test.

282. The answer is e. (*Rakel, pp 268–272.*) Any of the conditions listed as answers in this question can cause an exudative pharyngitis. Palatal petechiae suggest either a group A streptococcal infection of Epstein–Barr virus (EBV) pharyngitis. However, posterior cervical adenopathy should point to EBV as the correct diagnosis.

283. The answer is d. *(Rakel, pp 268–272.)* Fever, chills, myalgias, and pain with swallowing are nonspecific signs, and are associated with pharyngitis from any cause. Anterior adenopathy is also associated with viral or bacterial pharyngitis. However, uveal edema is suggestive of group A hemolytic streptococcal infection. First line treatment should be amoxicillin, as up to 15% of group A streptococcal infections are resistant to penicillin. Doxycycline can be a good second-line agent. Macrolides are not generally effective, as they have poor penetration and may induce resistance.

284. The answer is b. *(Rakel, pp 268–272.)* Approximately 30% of patients with infectious mononucleosis are colonized with group A streptococcal organisms. Therefore, their rapid streptococcal antigen and throat cultures may be positive. When patients with mononucleosis are treated with penicillin or amoxicillin, they often develop a maculopapular skin rash that may be confused with scarlet fever. The distinguishing feature in this case is posterior chain adenopathy, consistent with an infectious mononucleosis.

285. The answer is e. *(Rakel, pp 268–272.)* The best antibiotics to eliminate group A streptococcal carriage from oropharyngeal secretions are an oral respiratory quinolone or oral clindamycin. The other therapies would be less likely to eliminate colonization.

286. The answer is a. *(Rakel, pp 268–272.)* Laryngitis with pharyngitis is generally associated with a viral infection, and only supportive care is needed. Antibiotic therapy is not indicated in this case.

287. The answer is a. *(Rakel, pp 947–949.)* Acne is associated with many myths regarding its cause. The true cause is multifactorial, but likely related to disturbances of keratinization, hormonal secretion, and immune response. Acne is not caused by dirt, diet, or oily hair on the forehead. Interestingly stress does likely play a role, but even then, just a small role.

288. The answer is a. *(Rakel, pp 947–949.)* The central lesion in acne is the microcomedo. Therefore most acne treatment plans should involve a keratolytic. Retinoids are excellent keratolytics, and may be used as monotherapy in many cases, with the patients understanding that resolution may take months. Topical erythromycin and clindamycin have become less useful as monotherapy, as there has been a dramatic increase in resistance of *Propionibacterium acnes* to the antibiotics alone. The addition of benzoyl peroxide to the regimen effectively prevents resistance. Oral antibiotics may work, but cephalosporins should not be used. The medications of choice include erythromycins, tetracyclines trimethoprim-sulfamethoxazole, and ciprofloxacin. Oral contraceptives can often be used as an adjunct treatment in women, but most people would not use it as a first line agent. Topical steroids can be occasionally helpful, but invariably cause atrophy of the facial skin if used for too long.

289. The answer is b. *(Rakel, pp 947–949.)* Worsening acne in its most severe form is acne fulminans. It must be avoided, as it is especially vicious and leads to significant scarring. Many families have heard that depression is a significant side effect of isotretinoin, but large studies have failed to note any correlation. Dry skin and joint aches are side effects, but shouldn't warrant discontinuing the medication unless intolerable. Pregnancy is not a side effect of medication, but if it were to occur during the treatment, it would warrant discontinuation. Because of the teratogenicity associated with isotretinoin, women taking the medication must use two forms of birth control—one hormonal and one barrier. A pregnancy test must be obtained monthly, and treatment continued only if it is negative.

290. The answer is b. *(Rakel, pp 947–949.)* The patient in the picture has rosacea. Although it is often considered along with acne, rosacea is a distinct entity. Comedo formation, the hallmark of acne vulgaris, is absent in rosacea. About 50% of the patients with rosacea have eye involvement, including styes, blepharitis, and corneal surface disease. Topical steroids should be avoided, as they ultimately make the disease worse. Oral tetracyclines are useful—isotretinoin is the last resort. Treatments aimed at reducing the colonization of *P. acnes* without an anti-inflammatory treatment arm are not effective.

291. The answer is c. *(Rakel, pp 953–962.)* The patient shown above has a classic nodular basal cell carcinoma, the most common type of basal cell cancer. It is characterized as a shiny papule, generally with a depressed central keratotic plug and visible telangiectasia near the border. Verruca do not generally have the depressed center or the pearly borders. Molluscum can look similar, but usually do not have the visible telangiectasia present. Squamous cell cancers generally have a scale and the absence of classic BCC features. Cutaneous T-cell lymphoma have a variable presentation, usually with patches, plaques or tumors, and would be difficult to diagnosis by site alone.

292. The answer is e. *(Rakel, pp 962–970.)* The patient pictured has psoriasis. Topical corticosteroids are the most common therapeutic agents used to treat psoriasis. There is no place for antibiotics in treatment, except in the case of guttate psoriasis, a form that follows streptococcal infection and appears as multiple teardrops that erupt abruptly. Elidel is used for eczema, and although some use it to treat psoriasis, it is currently an off-label use. While the topical retinoid tazarotene (Tazorac) can be used, vitamin A is not indicated.

293. The answer is b. *(Rakel, pp 962–970.)* Dovonex is a vitamin-D derived analogue that includes epidermal differentiation and inhibits keratinocyte proliferation. The answer c refers to topical retinoid therapy, while the answer d refers to tacrolimus. Salicylic acid is described as a topical keratolytic.

294. The answer is a. *(Rakel, pp 962–970.)* The rash shown is classic for pityriasis rosea, a self-limited papulosquamous eruption. The treatment includes antihistamines or corticosteroids to relieve itch. There is no role for the other agents listed.

295. The answer is b. *(Rakel, pp 1006–1010.)* The child shown has impetigo. This diagnosis should be considered in the face of well-demarcated erythematous lesions that, when disrupted, develop a secondary golden crust. The lesions have a predilection for traumatized skin, in this case where nasal discharge has disrupted the skin surface. In the past, most cases were thought to be due to streptococci. However, most cases are caused by *S. aureus*.

296. The answer is a. *(Rakel, pp 1006–1010.)* The patient described and shown has "hot tub folliculitis." The infection is generally caused by *Pseudomonas aeruginosa* or *Pseudomonas cepacia*. However, the condition is usually self-limited. Antibiotic therapy is not indicated, except in recalcitrant cases, and usually reassurance is all that is necessary.

297. The answer is d. *(Rakel, pp 1010–1017.)* The description and picture are consistent with a recurrence of herpes simplex virus infection. Symptomatic primary infections are characterized by gingivostomatitis with or without cutaneous or perioral lesions. Fever, malaise, and tender adenopathy are common with primary infections. Recurrences are usually less severe. The episode shown above is a recurrence because it appears as grouped vesicles as opposed to gingivostomatitis. There is no way to differentiate HSV-1 from HSV-2 simply by looking at the lesions. Lesions are sometimes mistaken for bacterial processes because they can be pustular. Triggers for recurrences are ultraviolet light exposure or illness.

298. The answer is e. *(Rakel, pp 1010–1017.)* Treatment options for genital herpes include treating each outbreak or using chronic suppressive therapy to prevent outbreaks. Daily therapy decreases the rate of asymptomatic viral shedding and significantly reduces the number of reoccurrences. In the past, it was reserved for those with frequent infections, but recent evidence suggests that most people with HSV-2 infections use suppressive therapy. There is no single-dose therapy that has been shown to be effective. Weekly dosing is not indicated.

299. The answer is b. *(Rakel, pp 1010–1017.)* The patient shown has herpes zoster, or "shingles." Antiviral therapy is the treatment of choice, and can decrease the time for lesion healing and shorten the overall duration of pain if initiated within 72 hours after the onset. In some cases, no benefit will occur if treatment starts after the 72 hour cutoff, but it should be initiated regardless of time in patients over 50, those who are immunosuppressd, or those with eye involvement. Corticosteroids have not been shown to decrease the likelihood of postherpetic neuralgia. No antiviral is clearly superior to another. Antiviral resistance is actually uncommon in this setting.

300. The answer is b. *(Rakel, pp 1010–1017.)* The picture shown, coupled with the clinical scenario described, is classic for infection with Parvovirus B19. The resulting illness is called erythema infectiosum, or "fifth disease." Enteroviruses may cause hand-foot-and-mouth disease. Parainfluenza viruses are implicated in croup. Varicella causes chicken pox, and cytomegalovirus may cause mono-like symptoms, but not the classic "slapped cheek" appearing rash.

301. The answer is d. *(Rakel, pp 1021–1025.)* The picture shows tinea capitis. Systemic therapy is necessary for a cure, but concurrent use of topical ketoconazole shampoo or selenium sulfide lotion may kill spores on the hair. Griseofulvin is FDA approved for this indication, but fluconazole is not.

302. The answer is c. *(Rakel, pp 1021–1025.)* Tinea corporis, otherwise called "ringworm" is usually caused by *Trichophyton rubrum*. It appears as a well-demarcated plaque with central scaling. It is usually pruritic. Pityriasis rosea begins with a herald patch and develops as finer diffuse lesions.

Psoriasis is generally found on the extensor surfaces of the skin, and would be unlikely to appear for the first time in this manner. Atopic dermatitis usually appears on the flexural surfaces of the body, and is less likely to have the raised borders seen in this picture. Contact dermatitis is usually vesicular.

303. The answer is e. *(Mengel, pp 332–338.)* The symptoms in this case are consistent with viral conjunctivitis. The presence of a palpable preauricular lymph node is characteristic of viral conjunctivitis. Approximately 85% of viral conjunctivitis is due to adenovirus, which is highly contagious, and is self-limited. Only 15% of conjunctivitis is bacterial. Characteristics of bacterial conjunctivitis include purulent discharge, pain, photophobia, and a "gritty" sensation of the eye. Topical corticosteroids are contraindicated in conjunctivitis, as studies have documented increased duration of viral shedding, prolongation of the infectious period, and potential corneal ulcerations and perforations. Antiviral eye drops are indicated for herpetic eye infections, but without corneal dendrites with fluorescein staining, that diagnosis is unlikely. The treatment for nonherpetic viral conjunctivitis is supportive, using cold compresses and lubricating drops.

304. The answer is a. *(Mengel, pp 332–338.)* Gonorrheal infection of the eye is a medical emergency. Left untreated, it can lead to corneal ulceration or perforation within 24 hours. Chlamydial conjunctivitis needs to be treated, but does not require immediate ophthalmologic referral for evaluation. Corneal abrasions can be treated by a family physician, with the goal of pain control and rapid healing assistance. Subconjunctival hemorrhages are due to the spontaneous rupture of small subconjunctival vessels, and are easily treated in the outpatient setting. Blepharitis is a commonly seen inflammation of the eyelids, often due to seborrhea.

305. The answer is e. *(Rakel, pp 230–233.)* Symptoms of conjunctivitis include increased redness, irritation, tearing, discharge, photophobia or itching. Pain is more suggestive of a more serious problem, possibly a corneal abrasion or other pathology.

306. The answer is e. *(Rakel, pp 230–233.)* Of the symptoms of conjunctivitis, itching is more specific for allergic conditions. The other things listed (except for use of oral contraceptives) are more general and not useful in differentiating allergic conjunctivitis from other causes. The use of oral contraceptives may, in some people, cause a dry eye, but is less likely to cause conjunctivitis.

307. The answer is c. *(Rakel, pp 230–233.)* Adenovirus is the most common virus causing conjunctivitis. It can be transmitted through ocular and respiratory secretions, and less commonly from fomites on towels or equipment. It has an 8-day incubation period, and a 10–12 day viral shedding period. Supportive treatment is indicated.

308. The answer is d. *(Rakel, pp 230–233.)* Bacterial conjunctivitis is most commonly caused by *Streptococcus* and *Staphylococcus*. However, gram-negative organisms should be strongly suspected in contact lens wearers. Therefore, gentamicin is the medication of choice. If gram-negative organisms are not suspected, fluoroquinolones or polymyxin-trimethoprim can be used.

309. The answer is e. *(Mengel, pp 332–338. Rakel, pp 230–233.)* Gonococcal conjunctivitis is considered an ophthalmologic emergency because of this organism's propensity to cause corneal perforation. The patient will have a red, irritated eye with copious purulent discharge. After cleaning the eye, it reforms almost immediately. Initial therapy would include intravenous ceftriaxone along with topical fluoroquinolone or tobramycin therapy. One should also consider concurrent treatment for chlamydial conjunctivitis.

310. The answer is a. *(Rakel, pp 230–233.)* Scleritis is a unilateral diffuse injection of the deeper scleral vessels. Symptoms include decreased vision, deep "boring" eye pain and a surrounding headache. It is usually associated with systemic autoimmune diseases like rheumatoid arthritis or Wegener's granulomatosis. Episcleritis is associated with mild irritation, and is not as intense as the syndrome described above. A corneal abrasion is associated with decreased vision, intense pain, and tearing, but is associated with trauma. Acute glaucoma is associated with pain, decreased vision and redness, but the affected pupil is usually dilated. Iritis also has similar symptoms, but the pupil is small.

311. The answer is e. *(Rakel, pp 255–258.)* Despite the fact that rhinosinusitis is the most commonly reported chronic condition reported on health surveys, and despite the fact that it accounts for approximately 12% of all antibiotics prescribed in the United States, there is no specific sign or symptom that defines sinusitis. The most common symptoms are congestion, facial pressure, nasal discharge, dental pain, loss of smell, and headache. Persistence of symptoms beyond the usual 7–10 day course of a viral upper respiratory infection most commonly defines clinical rhinosinusitis.

312. The answer is a. *(Rakel, pp 255–258.)* While all of the conditions listed predispose to bacterial infections of the sinus cavities, allergic rhinitis is the most common one listed. It is present in at least 60% of people with recurrent sinusitis.

313. The answer is d. *(Rakel, pp 255–258.)* *Streptococcus pneumoniae* and nontypable *H. influenzae* are the most commonly cultured organisms in radiographically documented acute sinusitis. *Moraxella catarrhalis* is cultured from approximately 20% of pediatric cases, but is more uncommon in adults. *S. aureus* can be cultured from approximately 30% of healthy noses, but is uncommonly cultured in specimens obtained from acute sinusitis. Chronic sinusitis is more commonly polymicrobial.

314. The answer is d. *(Rakel, pp 255–258.)* Chronic sinusitis is classically defined as symptoms that persist beyond 3 months. However, the more common history is that of symptoms that improve with therapy then reoccur. In general, empirical therapy of adult chronic sinusitis should begin with fluoroquinolones or amoxicillin/clavulanate for 2–3 weeks. High dose amoxicillin or a cephalosporin may also be considered, but for 14–21 days.

315. The answer is d. *(Rakel, pp 255–258.)* Decongestants such as phelylpropanolamine and pseudoephedrine have not been shown to change the course of clinical respiratory tract disease. Alpha agonists have not been shown to shorten the course of sinusitis, and can lead to symptomatic rebound congestion after just 1 week of use. Echinacea has not been shown to prevent or to speed resolution of sinusitis. Topical nasal steroids are the most potent treatment for nasal congestion and have been shown to potentiate the treatment benefits of antibiotics in chronic sinusitis.

316. The answer is a. *(Rakel, pp 1218–1222.)* The injury described is called a "burner" or "stinger." They are very common in contact sports, and usually are sustained by a lateral flexion force distracting the head and shoulder away from the affected side, compression injury with the head and neck flexed toward the affected side, or a direct blow to the supraclavicular region. If symptoms resolve, and neck palpation and range of motion, shoulder and upper extremity neurological examination are all normal, patients can return to play. If both sides are involved, radiographs should be obtained to rule out cervical spine injury. An electromyography (EMG) can be obtained, but may take up to 3 weeks after the injury to become abnormal. Physical therapy may be useful for residual symptoms.

317. The answer is e. (*Rakel, pp 1218–1222.*) The injury described above is a type IV acromioclavicular separation. This is defined by more than a 50% separation of the joint with a posterior displacement of the clavicle. Treatment should be surgical. With less severe separations, treatment can be conservative—with sling immobilization, early range of motion exercises—and return to play when the pain subsides.

318. The answer is d. (*Rakel, pp 1218–1222.*) The patient described has patellofemoral syndrome, the most common overuse injury seen in the athlete under 40 years of age. While the mechanism is poorly understood, it is felt to be due to biomechanics, with the patella tracking laterally to the more developed vastus lateralis muscle. Patients complain of knee pain with use, but also note pain when the knee is held in flexion for long periods of time (the "movie theatre sign"). Treatment should be directed at stretching the hamstrings and building the vastus medialis muscle to improve biomechanics.

319. The answer is b. (*Rakel, pp 1218–1222.*) The twisting injury, feeling of a "pop" and immediate effusion while still being able to bear weight are consistent with an ACL tear. The sense of instability also helps lead toward that diagnosis. Patellofemoral pain would generally not occur acutely or after an injury. The mechanism of a posterior cruciate ligament injury is through direct force to the knee. Meniscal injuries also cause knee pain, but are more likely to cause locking, catching or giving way. Collateral ligament tears would likely lead to more instability than that described above.

320. The answer is d. (*Rakel, pp 1218–1222.*) The test described is McMurray's test, and is positive when the maneuver elicits a catch or click with pain at the joint line, indicating a meniscal tear.

321. The answer is a. (*Rakel, pp 1218–1222.*) The Ottawa ankle rules are a useful guide to use to determine if radiographs are indicated after an ankle sprain. Films should be obtained if:
- The patient is unable to walk four steps immediately after the injury and in the office
- There is tenderness over the distal 6 cm of the tibia or fibula, including the malleoli
- There is mid-foot or navicular tenderness
- There is tenderness over the proximal fifth metatarsal

Rest, ice, compression, and elevation are mainstays of therapy, but the x-ray is imperative for this case. Early mobilization is recommended, unless there is a fracture present. NSAIDs should be reserved for 48 hours after an injury because it may exacerbate bleeding and swelling acutely. Physical therapy may help expedite return to activity in the long run, but only after fracture has been ruled out.

322. The answer is c. (*Mengel, pp 359–364.*) Syncope can be classified as neurally mediated (vasovagal syncope, situational syncope), cardiac (arrhythmia or structurally related), cerebrovascular (transient ischemic attack [TIA], stroke, vertebrobasilar insurriciency, or subclavian steal syndrome), other differentiated (psychiatric causes) or idiopathic cause (unknown cause). Up to 50% of syncope is neurally mediated, and up to 23% are cardiac in origin. Cardiac syncope has a higher mortality rate than all other etiologies combined (20–30% at 1 year versus 6% for all other causes).

323. The answer is c. (*Mengel, pp 359–364.*) Studies have shown that a limited evaluation including a hematocrit, serum creatine kinase, glucose, ECG, carotid massage, orthostatic blood pressure and evaluation of pulses yields a diagnosis of syncope in the majority of cases. Additional testing including a Holter monitor, echocardiogram, ambulatory loop ECG, and tilt table testing yields a diagnosis in an additional 5% of patients. All patients with syncope should have an ECG, even though the diagnostic yield is low. It is relatively easy, risk-free, and can help rule out the most concerning cardiac causes. A CBC (including white blood cell count and platelets) is probably not needed unless an infectious etiology is suspected, and a thyroid stimulating hormone is also not necessary unless thyroid disease is suspected.

324. The answer is a. (*Mengel, pp 359–364.*) In syncopal patients who present with a heart murmur, echocardiography should be obtained. It will help rule out valvular heart disease, but will also identify hypertrophic cardiomyopathy (the likely cause in this question). Holter monitoring and long-term ambulatory loop ECG testing will help identify arrhythmias, stress testing will help identify ischemia and/or exercise induced arrhythmias, and tilt table tests are indicated in patients with unexplained recurrent syncope in whom cardiac causes are ruled out.

325. The answer is d. (*Mengel, pp 359–364.*) The patient in this scenario had exertional dyspnea and diaphoresis. As a diabetic, she is at high risk for silent ischemia, often signaled by anginal equivalents such as dyspnea and diaphoresis. A hypoglycemic event could have also caused diaphoresis and syncope, but serum glucose testing 1 day later would not help identify that as a cause. In addition, glycosolated hemoglobin would not be helpful in determining the cause of the event. An echocardiogram would not be helpful without physical examination findings consistent with cardiomyopathy or valvular disease, and a Holter monitor would be less helpful without evidence of palpitations or ECG abnormalities.

326. The answer is e. *(Mengel, pp 359–364.)* Tilt table testing is recommended in patients with unexplained recurrent syncope in whom cardiac causes including arrhythmias have been ruled-out. An abnormal result suggests vasovagal syncope. Psychiatric evaluation should be considered if the tilt table is normal, especially if associated with other psychiatric symptoms (anxiety, depression, fear, or dread). Carotid Dopplers and MRI of the brain should be reserved for people with bruits or focal neurological signs. Stress testing is indicated if there is high risk for, or symptoms of ischemic disease.

327. The answer is a. *(Taylor, pp 867–873.)* Contact and chemical dermatitidies can occur from the use of any topical agent in the genital area. Condoms and spermacides are common causes. The condition is characterized by a clear exudate and a reddened, swollen vulva or vaginal mucosa. Mycotic disease, trichomoniasis, and bacterial vaginosis would be unlikely to present with clear discharge, and chlamydia would be unlikely given the history and physical findings. While presentation is an important component of the diagnostic workup, laboratory testing, including saline and KOH preparations are critical in the evaluation of any vaginal discharge.

328. The answer is b. *(Taylor, pp 867–873.)* The classic presentation of vaginal candidiasis is vaginal itch with a white "cheesy" exudates. White plaques usually adhere to the vaginal wall. The KOH preparation shows multiple hyphae. Treatment consists of topical azole applications or an oral one-time dose of fluconazole. To date, no data prove oral medications to be superior to topical medications.

329. The answer is c. *(Taylor, pp 867–873.)* Recurrent yeast infections have been erroneously ascribed to many causes. They probably do NOT occur more frequently in diabetic women, but may be more difficult to eradicate in this population. Similarly, women with HIV may manifest or present with diffuse candidiasis that is difficult to eradicate, but not with recurrent infections. There is no convincing evidence that birth control pills cause infections. High calorie diets and crude fiber have been associated with susceptibility to infection. Although not a true sexually transmitted disease, when a patient has frequent relapses of vaginal candidiasis, treatment of the partner may achieve full eradication.

330. The answer is c. *(Taylor, pp 867–873.)* The history and physical described are classic for trichomonas vaginalis. The classic "strawberry cervix" is a strong diagnostic clue. Trichomonads are seen on high power in the saline preparation, and appear as triangular cells with long tails, slightly larger than white blood cells. "Studded" epithelial cells (clue cells) are more consistent with bacterial vaginosis, "Moth-eaten" cells (pseudo-clue cells) are seen in an acid-base disturbance of the vagina. Numerous white blood cells are more consistent with an upper genital infection, and hyphae are consistent with vaginal candidiasis.

331. The answer is a. *(Taylor, pp 867–873.)* The condition described is bacterial vaginosis. Clue cells, epithelial cells studded with bacteria, are diagnostically helpful. The treatment of choice is topical or oral metronidazole, with oral or topical clindamycin being an acceptable alternative. Doxycycline is used to treat chlamydia. Clotrimazole is used to treat fungal infections. Imiquimod is an immunomodulating agent approved to treat human papillomavirus infection, and acyclovir treats herpetic infections.

332. The answer is a. *(Mengel, pp 396–400.)* Acute viral respiratory tract infections cause up to 50% of wheezing episodes in children less than 2 years of age. Risk factors include fall or winter season, history of atopy, day care attendance and passive smoke exposure. Pneumonia causes 33–50% of wheezing episodes in children, and most are also caused by viruses as well. Bronchiolitis accounts for less than 5% of all episodes of wheezing, but is important, especially in preterm infants. Aspiration is uncommon, and is less likely in the setting of viral infection symptoms. Asthma is common in children, but is not diagnosed after one episode of wheezing.

333. The answer is d. *(Mengel, pp 396–400.)* Wheezing is commonly heard in patients with CHF. Risk factors include hypertension, glucose intolerance, and smoking. Treatment should begin with diuresis. Antibiotics would be prescribed for an infection, epinephrine for a suspected allergic reaction, steroids for an asthma exacerbation, and anticoagulation if a PE is suspected.

334. The answer is c. *(Mengel, pp 396–400.)* When a patient presents with acute shortness of breath and an increased respiratory rate, a PE must be ruled out. The patient in this case is taking oral contraceptives, increasing her risk for PE. An allergic reaction would likely cause an abnormal lung examination, and the other answer choices are more likely to occur insidiously.

335. The answer is b. *(Mengel, pp 396–400.)* Patients with a first episode of wheezing require a chest x-ray. Peak flow testing may be helpful in monitoring control of asthma, but are not useful in evaluating a first episode. Pulmonary function testing and a blood count may be needed, but a chest x-ray is an absolute necessity.

336. The answer is e. *(Mengel, pp 396–400.)* The patient described likely has gastroesophageal reflux, a common cause of wheezing in the pediatric population. The gold standard test is a 24 hour pH probe. Endoscopy is invasive, requires sedation, and is usually reserved for patients unresponsive to medical management. A chest x-ray is unlikely to reveal the cause in this case, and a barium swallow is indicated if the physician is concerned about structural defects. Pulmonary function testing is difficult in this age group.

337. The answer is b. *(Mengel, pp 396–400.)* In patients with known asthma, chest x-rays are not required to evaluate each episode. A chest x-ray is indicated if the patient has fever, rhonchi, or sputum to rule out pneumonia. Peak flows do not confirm the diagnosis of asthma, but are useful to monitor the status of known lung disease. Pulmonary function tests may be needed, but are usually done in a pulmonary laboratory. A blood count may indicate infection, but would be less useful in this setting. Nasopharyngeal washes may be helpful in the pediatric population, but are not as helpful for adults.

Chronic Conditions

Questions

338. A 46-year-old man is seeing you for help with smoking cessation. In addition to this, he reports having some sexual concerns. He complains of being unable to achieve erection, despite having strong interest in sexual activity. Which of the following is true regarding disorders of this sexual response phase?

a. Overcoming this disorder may require more visual stimulation
b. Overcoming this disorder may require more emphasis on the relationship
c. Overcoming this disorder requires an intact parasympathetic nervous system
d. Overcoming this disorder requires an intact sympathetic nervous system
e. Overcoming this disorder requires the use of androgens

339. A 36-year-old sees you to discuss a lack of sexual interest. He is not having sexual fantasies and is unmotivated to begin sexual activity. He does not report depressive symptoms and has no other physical complaints. His physical examination is normal. Which of the following laboratory tests is most appropriate?

a. Total testosterone
b. Free testosterone
c. Thyroid stimulating hormone
d. Prolactin
e. Prostate specific antigen

340. You are caring for a 45-year-old man with hypertension, gastroesophageal reflux, and depression. His medication list includes hydrochlorothiazide, verapamil, terazosin, omeprazole, bupropion, and trazodone. He is complaining of ejaculatory dysfunction. Which of the medications is most likely to cause this problem?

a. Hydrochlorothiazide
b. Verapamil
c. Terazosin
d. Omeprazole
e. Bupropion

341. You have diagnosed a 30-year-old woman with depression. She is concerned that medical treatment may cause sexual dysfunction. Which of the following antidepressants is least likely to cause sexual dysfunction?

a. Amitriptyline
b. Paroxetine
c. Citalopram
d. Sertraline
e. Bupropion

342. A 26-year-old newlywed man comes to your office to discuss premature ejaculation. He has had this condition since beginning sexual activity at 17 years old. He has tried behavioral methods, but these have not been successful. Which of the following medications is most likely to help this condition?

a. Alprostadil
b. Fluoxetine
c. Bupropion
d. Silendafil
e. Atenolol

343. You are seeing a 61-year-old patient and are concerned about substance abuse. He is single, employed as a lawyer in an extremely high stress job. Which of the characteristics listed below are known to increase his risk for a substance use disorder?

a. His age
b. His marital status
c. His job as a lawyer
d. His job stress
e. His level of education

344. You are evaluating a 31-year-old man who is concerned about depression. He reports depressed mood, increased irritability, anhedonia, and sleep and appetite disturbances for 3–4 weeks. He reports a long history of alcohol use, and is currently drinking 6 drinks a day on the weekdays, up to 12 on the weekends. His laboratory results are consistent with alcohol abuse. Which of the following is the most appropriate next step?

a. Treat with a selective serotonin reuptake inhibitor
b. Treat with bupropion
c. Recommend detoxification and abstinence

d. Recommend detoxification and abstinence and start a selective serotonin reuptake inhibitor

e. Recommend detoxification and abstinence and start bupropion

345. You suspect that a 50-year-old female patient is abusing alcohol. Which of the following is the most sensitive laboratory test to confirm this?

a. Mean corpuscular volume (MCV)
b. Alanine aminotransferase (ALT)
c. Aspartate aminotransferase (AST)
d. Gamma-glutamyl transferase (GGT)
e. Lactate dehydrogenase (LDH)

346. An alcoholic patient of yours is interested in pharmacologic therapy to help him in his sobriety. His counselor recommended he try naltrexone, and he asks you how that medication works in alcoholism. Which of the following is the best answer for your patient?

a. If the person taking naltrexone ingests alcohol, it causes an adverse reaction
b. Naltrexone reduces the reinforcing effects of alcohol
c. Naltrexone blocks the effects of alcohol by binding to alcohol receptor sites on cells
d. Naltrexone saturates the alcohol receptor sites on cells by acting as an alcohol agonist
e. Naltrexone changes the binding sites on alcohol, making it unable to bind to cells

347. An alcoholic patient of yours is interested in pharmacologic therapy to help him in his sobriety. His counselor recommended he try disulfiram, and he asks you how that medication works in alcoholism. Which of the following is the best answer for your patient?

a. If the person taking disulfiram ingests alcohol, it causes an adverse reaction
b. Disulfiram reduces the reinforcing effects of alcohol
c. Disulfiram blocks the effects of alcohol by binding to alcohol receptor sites on cells
d. Disulfiram saturates the alcohol receptor sites on cells by acting as an alcohol agonist
e. Disulfiram changes the binding sites on alcohol, making it unable to bind to cells

348. A 33-year-old male patient is seeing you for advice on how to quit smoking. He has tried many times in the past and has been unsuccessful. Which of the following symptoms characterize the nicotine withdrawal syndrome?

a. Hypersomnolence
b. Depressed mood
c. Psychomotor retardation
d. Lethargy
e. Amotivational syndrome

349. A 25-year-old woman is trying to stop smoking. She has difficulty with sudden cravings for nicotine and wonders which nicotine replacement system offers the fastest delivery of nicotine. Which of the following methods of nicotine replacement delivers nicotine fastest?

a. Nicotine gum
b. Nicotine lozenges
c. Transdermal nicotine patch
d. Nicotine nasal spray
e. Nicotine inhaler

350. One of your patients has tested positive for cocaine use. Upon questioning, he says he would like to quit, but has a difficult time with cocaine withdrawal. Which of the following symptoms is expected from cocaine withdrawal?

a. Tachycardia
b. Hypertension
c. Depression
d. Anxiety
e. Insomnia

351. You are caring for a 35-year-old man in the hospital, admitted with pneumonia. On day 2 of his hospitalization, he becomes diaphoretic, restless, and irritable. Within hours, he is complaining of severe pain, abdominal cramps, and diarrhea. Which of the following would likely be present in his urine toxicology screen?

a. Cocaine
b. Marijuana
c. Opiates
d. 3,4-Methylenedioxymethampheatmine (MDMA or ecstasy)
e. Benzodiazepines

352. A 64-year-old woman comes to see you as a new patient. She is interested in finding the cause of her hand deformities. Upon inspection, you see the joints in her hands are nodular and enlarged as in the picture below:

(Reproduced, with permission, from South-Paul J. Current Diagnosis & Treatment in Family Medicine, *1st ed. New York: McGraw-Hill, 2004:266.)*

Which of the following laboratory findings is likely in her case?

a. Her laboratory evaluation will likely be normal
b. Her serum uric acid level will likely be elevated
c. Her sedimentation rate will likely be elevated
d. Her c-reactive protein level will likely be elevated
e. Her rheumatoid factor will likely be elevated

353. You are evaluating a 62-year-old man who is complaining of joint pain. His pain involves his left knee, right ankle, and both hands. He reports that his symptoms have been present for years, but are worsening. He has more pain with activity. On examination, you note some swelling in the joints with mild tenderness and crepitus. What is the likely cause of his symptoms?

a. Rheumatoid arthritis
b. Osteoarthritis
c. Gout
d. Tendonitis
e. Fibromyalgia

354. A 43-year-old obese patient comes to your office with a painful, inflamed, swollen elbow. He reports that the pain began suddenly last evening, without a known precipitant or trauma. The pain is exquisite, and does not allow him to move his elbow at all—in fact, even the pressure of his bed sheet on his elbow was painful. On examination, he has an elbow effusion with warmth, erythema, and intense pain with movement. Which of the following is most likely the cause?

a. Rheumatoid arthritis
b. Osteoarthritis
c. Gout
d. A stress fracture
e. Cellulitis

355. You are caring for a 31-year-old woman who complains of joint pain. She notes that her hands seem to be stiff in the morning, and that she seems to improve with time, movement, and heat. She reports more fatigue than usual as well. On examination, her wrists are swollen bilaterally, as are several of her metacarpal-phalangeal joints on each hand. Which of the following is her most likely diagnosis?

a. Rheumatoid arthritis
b. Osteoarthritis
c. Gout
d. Tendonitis
e. Fibromyalgia

356. A 70-year-old man with diabetes and long-term osteoarthritis in his knees is presenting for follow up. He reports that his pain has become much more severe, and says he is having difficulty with ambulation and actually becoming fairly inactive. In the past, he tried ibuprofen and naproxen, but those offered limited improvement and he developed secondary ulcers. He says that taking acetaminophen is like "taking a sugar pill"—and says it offers no help. He had some relief from steroid injections 3 months ago, and again 1 month ago, but they were short-lived. A recent x-ray is shown below:

Which of the following is the next most appropriate step in the treatment of his condition?

a. Use oral steroids
b. Try another steroid injection
c. Inject the knee joint with ketorolac (Toradol)
d. Inject hyaluronic acid into his knee joints
e. Refer for knee replacements

(Reproduced, with permission, from South-Paul J. Current Diagnosis & Treatment in Family Medicine, 1st ed. New York: McGraw-Hill, 2004:267)

357. You are seeing a 43-year-old man who complains of recurrent flares of gout. He notes that he gets "attacks" after drinking alcohol and asks why. Which of the following is the best response?

a. Alcohol causes the release of uric acid from the liver
b. Alcohol itself increases crystal formation in the joint
c. Alcohol alters renal excretion of uric acid
d. Alcohol contains relatively large quantities of uric acid
e. Alcohol contains sulfites that metabolize into uric acid after absorption in the gut

358. A 66-year-old diabetic man comes to your office with acute monoarticular arthritis. You suspect gout. Which of the following tests is the most helpful in establishing the diagnosis?

a. Sedimentation rate
b. C-reactive protein
c. Serum uric acid levels
d. Evaluation of joint aspirate
e. Twenty-four hour urine collection to measure uric acid excretion

359. You are evaluating a patient with knee swelling and pain. You perform an arthrocentesis to help determine the diagnosis. The fluid analysis reveals rhomboid-shaped positive birefringent crystals. Which of the following is the likely diagnosis?

a. Gout
b. Pseudogout
c. Infectious arthritis
d. Osteoarthritis
e. Rheumatoid arthritis

360. You are evaluating a patient with a painful, swollen knee. You perform arthrocentesis to find cloudy fluid. Analysis reveals a white blood cell count of 50,000 with more than 90% identified as polymorphonuclear leukocytes. The glucose level in the joint fluid is decreased. Which of the following is the most likely diagnosis?

a. Gout
b. Pseudogout
c. Infectious arthritis
d. Osteoarthritis
e. Rheumatoid arthritis

361. You are evaluating a patient with a painful, swollen knee. Joint aspirate reveals clear fluid with a white blood cell count of 5000, 20% of which are polymorphonuclear leukocytes. Which of the following is the most likely diagnosis?

a. Gout
b. Pseudogout
c. Infectious arthritis
d. Osteoarthritis
e. Rheumatoid arthritis

362. The joint aspirate from the inflamed first metatarsal phalangeal joint of a 35-year-old woman reveals needle-shaped nonbirefringent crystals. Which of the following is the most appropriate initial treatment?

a. Colchicine
b. Corticosteroids
c. Opiates
d. Allopurinol
e. Probenecid

363. You are following a 52-year-old woman with stiff, swollen hands. Her left hand is shown below:

(Reproduced, with permission, from South-Paul J. Current Diagnosis & Treatment in Family Medicine, *1st ed. New York: McGraw-Hill, 2004:276.)*

Her right hand is similar. She describes prolonged morning symptoms, and excessive fatigue. Based on this information, which of the following is the most likely diagnosis?

a. Osteoarthritis
b. Gout
c. Tophaceous gout
d. Rheumatoid arthritis
e. Systemic lupus erythematosis

364. You are caring for a 45-year-old woman who was diagnosed with rheumatoid arthritis 6 years ago. Which of the following signs or symptoms, if present, would signal extra-articular manifestations of her condition?

a. Cough
b. Palpitations
c. Gastrointestinal distress
d. Peripheral neuropathy
e. Elevated creatinine

365. You have recently determined that a patient in your office has rheumatoid arthritis. Which of the following is the most appropriate next step?

a. Control symptoms with nonsteroidal anti-inflammatory medications
b. Control symptoms with opiates
c. Use steroid treatment for flares, and nonsteroidal anti-inflammatory medications for daily use
d. Use steroid injections to keep flares under control
e. Refer to rheumatology

366. You are caring for a 35-year-old man with a long history of allergies and asthma. His asthma has been in good control, but his blood pressure has been elevated on more than two occasions despite weight loss, exercise and appropriate dietary intervention. Which of the following blood pressure medications should be avoided in this case?

a. Hydrochlorothiazide
b. Lisinopril (Zestril, Prinivil)
c. Nifedipine (Procardia)
d. Propranolol (Inderal)
e. Losartin (Cozaar)

367. You have recently diagnosed a 24-year-old man with asthma. You are discussing environmental measures he should take to control his symptoms and avoid triggers. Which of the following is the most appropriate advice?

a. Keep humidity in the home relatively high, above 50%
b. Enclose his mattress and pillows with allergen impermeable covers
c. Launder bed linens with cold water
d. Install carpeting if possible
e. Use air filters to decrease the levels of dust mite allergens

368. You are seeing a 19-year-old college student complaining of recurrent and persistent cough. She has been treated for "bronchitis" several times, and you are concerned that her true diagnosis is asthma. Which of the following is most important in the diagnosis of asthma?

a. History
b. Allergy testing
c. Chest x-ray
d. Pulmonary function tests with and without bronchodilator therapy
e. Provocative testing with methocholine

369. You are caring for a 30-year-old woman who has had asthma since childhood. Currently, she reports symptoms three or four times a week, but never more than once a day. Sometimes her symptoms cause her to skip her usual exercise regimen. She wakes in the night approximately three or four times a month to use her inhaler and return to bed. Which of the following classifications best characterizes her asthma?

a. Mild intermittent
b. Moderate intermittent
c. Mild persistent
d. Moderate persistent
e. Severe persistent

370. You are caring for an 18-year-old man with asthma. He smokes, and reports needing to use his short-acting bronchodilator daily. He gets flares of asthma at least twice a week, and while some days are relatively symptom free, some exacerbations may last several days. He wakes up at least once a week with symptoms. Which of the following classifications best characterizes his asthma?

a. Mild intermittent
b. Moderate intermittent
c. Mild persistent
d. Moderate persistent
e. Severe persistent

371. You are discussing asthma control with a 22-year-old patient. She monitors her therapy closely, and reports that her current peak flows are at about 80% of her best levels. Which of the following is the best approach to take at this point?

a. Commend the patient on her diligent monitoring and excellent control
b. Reassure the patient that this is well within the normal range
c. Review the patient's medications and technique and review environmental control
d. Have the patient take additional medication, or add a medication to her regimen
e. Consider hospitalization

372. You are caring for a young woman who has had mild intermittent asthma for years. She uses a short-acting bronchodilator as needed, but in the past has only needed therapy once or twice a month. Over the past 2 months, she has noted that she is using her inhaler more. In fact, she uses it at least three times a week, and on occasion has had to wake up in the middle of the night to use her inhaler. Of the following, which is the most appropriate treatment option at this point?

a. Change her short-acting beta-agonist from albuterol (Proventil, Ventolin) to pirbuterol (Maxair)
b. Add a long-acting beta-agonist
c. Add an inhaled corticosteroid
d. Add a leukotriene receptor antagonist
e. Add cromolyn (Intal)

373. You are caring for a man with asthma. He is currently taking an inhaled corticosteroid twice daily and using his short acting beta agonist as needed. Over the past 3 months, he has required escalating doses of his inhaled corticosteroid, and now he is at the maximum dosage, still using his "rescue" inhaler more than he would like. Of the following, which is the best medication to add to his regimen?

a. A burst and rapid taper of oral steroids
b. A long-acting beta-agonist
c. Cromolyn (Intal)
d. Ipratropium (Atrovent)
e. Theophylline

374. You are caring for a 25-year-old woman who has had mild intermittent asthma since she was a child. She uses a short acting bronchodilator as needed. Over the past 5 weeks, she has been using her inhaler up to four times a week, and has had to wake up in the middle of the night to use her inhaler twice. She tried inhaled corticosteroids, but was intolerant of the side effects. Of the following, which is the most appropriate treatment option for her?

a. A long-acting beta-agonist
b. A leukotriene receptor antagonist
c. Cromolyn (Intal)
d. Theophylline
e. Oral corticosteroids

375. A 22-year-old man is seeing you to discuss his low back pain. He is athletic and exercises regularly. He denies any inciting event, does not have pain with movement, and denies radiation of the pain. Given this information, what is the most likely diagnosis?

a. Spondylolisthesis
b. Low back strain
c. Degenerative osteoarthritis
d. Lumbar disk herniation
e. Neoplasm

376. You are performing a preparticipation physical examination on a 14-year-old girl interested in playing lacrosse. You note asymptomatic scoliosis. You obtain x-rays that reveal a 15% thoracic curve to the right. Which of the following is the most appropriate next step?

a. Referral to orthopedic specialist
b. Refer for a thoracic back brace
c. Reassure, and reexamine the patient yearly
d. Obtain repeat x-rays every 6 months
e. Obtain an MRI (magnetic resonance imaging)

377. You are seeing a 44-year-old woman who is complaining of low back pain. She reports that her symptoms began several months ago, and started gradually. The pain is worse in the morning, and is associated with stiffness. It gets better throughout the day and with activity. She denies radiation or neurological symptoms. Which of the following is the most likely cause?

a. Back strain
b. An inflammatory condition
c. Disk herniation
d. Compression fracture
e. Neoplasm

378. You are evaluating a generally healthy 33-year-old man with low back pain. The pain began yesterday, occurring suddenly while loading firewood in his truck. He reports that the pain radiates to his right leg. On examination, his range of motion is limited by pain. His lower extremity neurological examination is normal. When you lay the patient on his back and raise his fully extended leg by the heel, he reports pain below the knee at about 30° of elevation. What is the most likely diagnosis?

a. Back strain
b. An inflammatory condition
c. Disk herniation
d. Compression fracture
e. Neoplasm

379. A 41-year-old sedentary man presented to you 6 weeks ago with the acute onset of low back pain radiating to the left leg. His neurological examination at the time was normal, but he did not respond to conservative therapy. X-rays are normal. What is the most appropriate next step?

a. Flexion and extension radiographs
b. MRI
c. Electromyelography
d. Bone scan
e. A complete blood count and erythrocyte sedimentation rate

380. A 35-year-old woman presents to you with low back pain. It occurred suddenly when lifting her 6-year-old son yesterday. She has tried acetaminophen without relief. On examination, her range of motion is limited by pain, and she has tenderness to palpation of the lumbar paraspinal muscles. Which of the following would be the best treatment option?

a. Bed rest for three to five days
b. Spinal traction
c. Nonsteroidal anti-inflammatory agents and return to normal activity
d. Opiate analgesia and limited activities
e. Oral corticosteroids

381. Despite several months of conservative therapy including physical therapy, one of your 44-year-old male patients has had persistent low back pain. Which of the following interventions has been shown to be effective in the short term?

a. An individualized exercise program
b. Antidepressants
c. Steroid injections
d. Traction
e. Acupuncture

382. You are evaluating a 31-year-old man complaining of left-sided neck and upper-back pain. He reports worsening discomfort when he turns his head toward the left, with some paresthesias in his left upper extremity. On examination, when you rotate his head to the left and exert downward pressure on his head, it reproduces the pain and paresthesia. Which of the following is the most likely diagnosis?

a. Cervical strain
b. Cervical disk herniation
c. Toroticollis

d. Spondylosis
e. Osteoarthritis

383. A 60-year-old woman was the restrained driver in a motor vehicle accident yesterday. Today, she presents to you for evaluation. She reports neck and upper back pain. On examination, she does not have bony tenderness, but cannot rotate her head 45° to the right or left. Which of the following is the most appropriate next step in her evaluation?

a. Reassurance and nonsteroidal anti-inflammatory agents
b. Cervical spine x-rays
c. MRI
d. Bone scan
e. Dual energy X-ray absorptiometry (DEXA) scan

384. You are assessing a 59-year-old patient with an 80-pack-year history of smoking cigarettes. He stopped smoking 1 year ago. He reports a cough productive of white frothy sputum for the past 4 months. Reviewing his chart, you discover that he had a similar presentation last winter, with a cough that lasted more than 3 months. Given this information, what is his most likely diagnosis?

a. Asthma
b. Chronic bronchitis
c. Bronchiectasis
d. Emphysema
e. Recurrent pneumonia

385. You have been treating a 33-year-old woman for asthma for the last three years. She began with mild symptoms, but has become progressively more short of breath over the last year. She reports weight loss and significant dyspnea on exertion. She has never smoked, but her husband smokes in the home. Her maternal aunt was a smoker, and died of emphysema in her early 50s. Her chest x-ray reveals flattened diaphragms, a long, narrow heart cardiac silhouette, and increased retrosternal airspace on the lateral projection. Given this clinical picture and x-ray, what is the most likely consideration?

a. HIV with chronic lung infection
b. Congestive heart failure
c. Chronic bronchitis
d. Lung cancer due to passive exposure to cigarette smoking
e. Alpha 1-antitrypsin deficiency

386. You are caring for a 64-year-old former smoker who complains of increasing shortness of breath with exertion and sometimes at rest. You observe that he is somewhat "barrel-chested," he breathes with pursed lips, and leans forward resting on his elbows when sitting in your office. On examination, he has decreased breath sounds and distant heart sounds. You are concerned about chronic obstructive pulmonary disease (COPD) and order office spirometry. Which measurement is most sensitive to diagnose COPD?

a. Total lung capacity (TLC)
b. Forced vital capacity (FVC)
c. Forced expiratory volume in 1 second (FEV_1)
d. Forced expiratory flow rate over the interval from 25% to 75% of the total FVC ($FEF_{25-75\%}$)
e. FEV_1/FVC ratio

387. You have diagnosed a 59-year-old woman with emphysema. In addition to pulmonary rehabilitation and lifestyle changes, you would like to try medical therapy. What should be your first line therapy in this patient?

a. A short-acting beta-adrenergic agent (albuterol)
b. A long-acting beta-adrenergic agent (salmeterol)
c. An anticholinergic agent (ipratropium)
d. Theophylline
e. A corticosteroid

388. A 64-year-old man with known chronic obstructive pulmonary disease complains of increasing dyspnea despite therapy with ipratropium and a short-acting beta-adrenergic agent. You are considering the addition of theophylline. Which of the following is true of this medication?

a. It does not enhance bronchodilation when added to ipratropium and beta-agonists
b. It should be considered in patients with cor pulmonale
c. The therapeutic range is wide, and the toxicity is low
d. Renal disease is a contraindication to the use of theophylline
e. Smoking slows the rate of metabolism

389. You are seeing a patient in the office for the first time. She is a 68-year-old recently retired school teacher with diabetes and hypertension. She is overweight and does not exercise regularly. Which of the following is the best indicator of the presence of renal insufficiency in this patient?

a. Her body mass index
b. The presence of diabetes
c. The presence of hyptertension
d. Her calculated or estimated glomerular filtration rate
e. Her serum creatinine level

390. You are following a 45-year-old man with difficult to control diabetes. As such, you are monitoring his kidney function and are alert to changes suggesting the beginning of chronic renal insufficiency. Of the following, which would occur first in the setting of chronic renal failure?

a. Hyperkalemia
b. Hyponatremia
c. Hyperphosphatemia
d. A fall in plasma bicarbonate level
e. Anemia

391. You are following a 56-year-old patient who has been diagnosed with hypertension and diabetes for 4 years. He does fairly well with diet and exercise, and has remained compliant with his medications. Laboratory evaluation demonstrates a normal serum creatinine, no microalbuminuria, but a glomerular filtration rate (GFR) of 70 mL/minute. According to the National Kidney Foundation staging guidelines, what stage of renal failure does this represent?

a. Stage 0 renal failure
b. Stage 1 renal failure
c. Stage 2 renal failure
d. Stage 3 renal failure
e. Stage 4 renal failure

392. You are seeing a newly diagnosed hypertensive patient in your office. As you are considering appropriate therapy for this patient you note that his mother had renal failure from hypertension and was on dialysis. Which of the following medications should you consider for blood pressure management?

a. An aldosterone antagonist
b. An angiotensin-converting enzyme (ACE) inhibitor
c. A beta-blocker
d. A calcium-channel blocker
e. A alpha$_1$-blocker

393. You are seeing a hypertensive patient in you office. He is well-controlled with hydrochlorozide, and is seeing you for a routine evaluation. His blood pressure at the visit is 118/76. Laboratory evaluation reveals a normal creatinine and a GFR greater than 90 mL/minute, but he does have microalbuminuria. Which of the following interventions is indicated in this patient?

a. Commend him on his excellent control and make no changes
b. Work to achieve better blood pressure control through diet and exercise
c. Increase his hydrochlorothiazide dose
d. Add an ACE inhibitor
e. Check a glycosolated hemoglobin level

394. You are following a patient with hypertension and diabetes in your office. Despite good blood pressure and glycemic control, his GFR has started to decrease. GFR measurement was 74 mL/minute 3 months ago. At this visit, GFR is 55 mL/minute. Creatinine is within normal limits, and his serum potassium is 5.2 mmol/L (normal is up to 5.1 mmol/L). The patient denies any changes in urination or other problems. Which of the following is most appropriate at this stage?

a. See the patient more frequently, at least monthly
b. Increase his ACE inhibitor
c. Add diuretic therapy
d. Refer to a nephrologist
e. Refer to a transplant surgeon

395. You are seeing a 48-year-old man with known cirrhosis. He has several physical signs of his illness, including spider angiomata, palmar erythema, Dupuytren's contractures, gynecomastia, testicular atrophy, splenomegaly, and parotid gland enlargement. Which of his physical examination findings are more commonly seen in patients with nonalcoholic causes of cirrhosis?

a. Spider angiomata
b. Dupuytren's contractures
c. Testicular atrophy
d. Splenomegaly
e. Parotid gland enlargement

396. You are following a patient who is known to have primary biliary cirrhosis. You are following his liver function tests as indicators of disease severity and progression. Which of the following tests, if rising, is the poorest prognostic sign?

a. Aspartate aminotransferase (AST)
b. ALT
c. Gamma-glutamyl transpeptidase (GGT)
d. Alkaline phosphatase
e. Bilirubin

397. You are following a cirrhotic patient with ascites. On laboratory evaluation, you note that he is hyponatremic. Which of the following is the most likely cause of his hyponatremia?

a. High levels of antidiuretic hormone secretion
b. Hepatic synthetic protein dysfunction causes osmotic losses of sodium
c. Shunting of blood away from the kidney to the liver
d. First pass excretion of sodium
e. Osmotic sodium shifts from the blood to the ascitic fluid

398. You are seeing a new patient. His history of alcohol use is significant, and he has several physical examination findings that are consistent with a potential diagnosis of cirrhosis. Which of the following is the best diagnostic test to confirm cirrhosis?

a. CT scan of the abdomen
b. Ultrasound of the abdomen
c. MRI of the abdomen
d. Radionuclide testing
e. Liver biopsy

399. You are evaluating a 48-year-old man with liver disease. His laboratory evaluation is as follows:

> AST: 298 u/L (H)
> ALT: 144 u/L (H)
> Alk Phos: 140 u/L (H)
> Bilirubin: 2.3 mg/dL (H)
> GGT: 220 u/L (H)

What is the most likely cause?

a. Autoimmune hepatitis
b. Hepatitis B
c. Hepatitis C
d. Hematochromatosis
e. Alcoholic hepatitis

400. You are evaluating a 45-year-old man with liver disease. His laboratory evaluation reveals the following:

AST: 52 u/L (H)
ALT: 56 u/L (H)
Alkaline phosphatase: 132 u/L (H)
GGT: 188 u/L (H)
Albumin: 2.9 g/dL (L)
Bilirubin: 3.5 mg/dL (H)
Prothrombin time: 14.9 sec (H)

Which of the following lab results is more likely to suggest chronic liver disease?

a. AST
b. ALT
c. GGT
d. Alkaline phosphatase
e. Albumin

401. You have just diagnosed a 46-year-old woman with cirrhosis. The patient also has asthma, arthritis, hypertension, depression, and hypothyroidism. Of the following, which medication should be avoided in this patient?

a. Albuterol
b. Nonsteroidal anti-inflammatory agents
c. Selective serotonin reuptake inhibitors
d. Angiotension converting enzyme inhibitors
e. Thyroid replacement

402. You are seeing a patient who has end-stage liver disease with cirrhosis due to hepatitis C. What will be her most likely cause of death?

a. Liver failure
b. Myocardial infarction
c. Bleeding varices
d. Hepatocellular carcinoma
e. Renal failure

403. You are taking care of a 47-year-old woman with cirrhosis. She asks you about transplantation as a definitive treatment option. Which of the following is an absolute contraindication to transplantation?

a. Active alcoholism
b. Portal vein thrombosis
c. Hepatitis B surface antigen positivity
d. Human immunodeficiency virus positivity
e. Extensive previous abdominal surgery

404. You are evaluating a 58-year-old man with coronary artery disease, hypertension and liver disease due to a history of alcoholism. He is presenting to you with shortness of breath, and on examination has hepatomegaly. To help determine the cause, you ask the patient to lie down, and while looking at his jugular veins, compress his right upper quadrant for 1 minute. If he has congestive heart failure, which of the following signs would you expect to see?

a. No change in the jugular veins during or immediately after right upper quadrant compression
b. Collapse of the jugular veins during and immediately after right upper quadrant compression
c. Collapse of the jugular veins during, but expansion of the veins immediately after right upper quadrant compression
d. Expansion of the jugular veins during and immediately after right upper quadrant compression
e. Expansion of the jugular veins during, but compression of the veins immediately after right upper quadrant compression

405. You are assessing a 54-year-old woman with suspected heart failure. You are auscultating her heart to listen for an S_3 gallop which you know to be a common finding in heart failure. Which of the following will give you the optimal chance of hearing a S_3 gallop?

a. Listening with the diaphragm of the stethoscope over the right sternal border with the patient squatting
b. Listening with the diaphragm of the stethoscope over the apical impulse with the patient in the left lateral decubitus position
c. Listening with the diaphragm of the stethoscope over the apical impulse with the patient standing
d. Listening with the bell of the stethoscope over the right sternal border with the patient squatting
e. Listening with the bell of the stethoscope over the apical impulse with the patient in the left lateral decubitus position

406. You are caring for a patient, who continues to smoke despite having asthma. She also has poorly controlled diabetes and hypertension with left ventricular hypertrophy. She presents to your office with shortness of breath. On physical examination, she appears to be in mild respiratory distress, and has 2+ pitting edema bilaterally. She has inspiratory and expiratory wheezes bilaterally, with dullness to percussion at the bases of her lungs. You order a stat b-type natriuretic peptide (BNP) and it comes back elevated at 498 pg/mL (normal is less than 100). Which of the following is the most likely diagnosis?

a. Asthma exacerbation
b. Pneumonia
c. Congestive heart failure
d. Pulmonary embolus
e. Aspiration

407. You have diagnosed a 66-year-old woman with heart failure. She has a history of hypertension, but has never had heart failure before. Which of the following tests is not routinely indicated?

a. An echocardiogram
b. A Holter monitor
c. Electrocardiogram
d. Complete blood count
e. Thyroid studies

408. You are seeing a patient in follow up after being hospitalized. She initially presented to the emergency room with dyspnea and was found to be in congestive heart failure. They admitted her for diuresis and initiation of appropriate first-line therapy. Since being released, she reports that she is comfortable at rest, but that ordinary activity results in mild dyspnea. According to the New York Heart Association Functional Classification, which class of heart failure best describes this patient?

a. Class I
b. Class II
c. Class III
d. Class IV
e. Class V

409. A 62-year-old woman comes to your office complaining of dyspnea. She has a history of chronic obstructive pulmonary disease, hypertension, and diabetes. She also smokes and drinks heavily. Her evaluation reveals that she is in heart failure. Which of the following interventions will lead to functional improvement in this patient?

a. Optimizing the treatment of her COPD
b. Optimizing the treatment of her hypertension
c. Optimizing her glycemic control
d. Discontinuing cigarette smoking
e. Discontinuing alcohol use

410. You have been treating a 61-year-old man for chronic heart failure. In his baseline state, he is comfortable at rest, but experiences some symptoms of heart failure with ordinary activity. You are having difficulty achieving optimal volume status using furosemide (Lasix) alone, and want to add another diuretic. Which of the following would be the best diuretic to add?

a. Hydrochlorothiazide
b. Triamterene
c. Hydrochlorothiazide and triamterene combined (Dyazide, Maxzide)
d. Metolazone (Zaroxolyn)
e. Spironolactone (Aldactone)

411. You have diagnosed a 49-year-old man with congestive heart failure due to left ventricular systolic dysfunction. In addition to acute diuresis, which of the following is the best first-line agent to use for treatment, in the absence of contraindications?

a. Angiotension converting enzyme inhibitors
b. Beta-blockers
c. Calcium-channel blockers
d. Nitrates
e. Hydralazine

412. After starting lisinopril for NYHA Class II heart failure due to left ventricular systolic dysfunction, a 69-year-old woman develops angioedema. Which of the following alternative therapies would be best for this patient?

a. Enalapril (Vasotec)
b. Losartin (Cozaar)
c. Nifedipine (Procardia, Adalat)
d. Metoprolol (Lopressor, Toprol)
e. Clonidine (Catapres)

413. You are treating a patient for heart failure due to systolic dysfunction with daily diuretics and an ACE inhibitor. He is continuing to have symptoms with activity, but they do not seem to be related to volume overload. Adding which of the following medications has been shown to reduce symptoms and improve mortality?

a. Metolazone (Zaroxolyn)
b. Spironolactone (Aldactone)
c. Metoprolol (Toprol XL)
d. Nifedipine (Procardia)
e. Digoxin (Lanoxin)

414. You take care of a 56-year-old woman whose 75-year-old mother just began living with her. The mother has been diagnosed with Alzheimer's disease. The daughter is trying to learn all she can about the illness and asks you what causes it. Which of the following is believed to be the critical pathologic problem involved in Alzheimer's disease?

a. Brain atrophy
b. Destruction of neurons
c. Edema of neurons
d. Shrinkage of large cortical neurons
e. Loss of synapses

415. Which of the following is the most consistent neurochemical change associated with Alzheimer's disease?

a. Deficiency in glutamate
b. Decline in cholinergic activity
c. Decreased norepinepherine levels
d. Increased somatostatin levels
e. Increased corticotrophin-releasing factor activity

416. You are concerned that one of your 65-year-old patients is developing dementia. Which of the following, if present, would lead you to suspect dementia rather than delirium or depression?

a. Acute onset of symptoms
b. Difficulty with concentration
c. Signs of psychomotor slowing
d. Good effort with testing, but wrong answers
e. Patient complaint of memory loss

417. You are caring for a 79-year-old woman with symptoms suggesting Alzheimer's disease. Which of the following clinical features of Alzheimer's disease is most likely to remain intact until the late stages of the disease?

a. The ability to recall new information
b. The amount of conversational output
c. The ability to draw complex figures (intersecting boxes or a clock)
d. The ability to calculate (balance a checkbook)
e. Appropriate social behavior

418. The daughter of one of your patients accompanies her mother to the office to discuss her concerns. The mother seems to have had progressive cognitive failure over the last year. According to the daughter, she loses function in a stepwise fashion. She seems to stabilize, but suddenly becomes less able to remember things or care for herself. This has happened several times in the last year. Given this history, what is the likely etiology of her dementia?

a. Alzheimer's disease
b. Parkinson's disease
c. Alcoholic dementia
d. Vascular dementia
e. Depression

419. You are concerned that a 66-year-old man is developing signs of Alzheimer's disease. His mother suffered from it, and he has an older brother currently battling dementia. Which of the following is considered a routine laboratory test used in the evaluation of dementia?

a. Erythrocyte sedimentation rate
b. Toxicology screening
c. Syphilis serology
d. An MRI of the brain
e. A heavy metal screen

420. You decide to treat a 72-year-old man for Alzheimer's dementia. You choose to use donepezil (Aricept), and begin therapy. Which of the following effects is *not* likely with the use of this medication?

a. Improvement in cognition
b. Improvement in behavior
c. Improvement in the ability to accomplish activities of daily living
d. Improvement in global measurements of functioning
e. Improvement in the progression of neurodegeneration

421. You are treating a patient with the classic signs of dementia. His caretaker reports that he has been having complex visual hallucinations and a tremor. On examination, he appears to have masked facies, has a slight tremor, and a shuffling gait. His cognitive decline is stable and present. Which of the following medications should be avoided in this case?

a. Cholinesterase inhibitors
b. Selective serotonin reuptake inhibitors
c. Tricyclic antidepressants
d. Antipsychotics
e. Benzodiazepines

422. You are performing a screening physical examination on a 47-year-old man. He is generally healthy, and his review of systems is negative. His mother has type 2 diabetes, and he is overweight. Which of the following is generally accepted as the test of choice to screen for type 2 diabetes?

a. A random glucose test
b. A fasting glucose
c. A urinalysis to screen for glycosuria
d. A 1-hour glucose tolerance test
e. A 3-hour glucose tolerance test

423. You are evaluating a 36-year-old obese woman who complains of fatigue. She denies polydipsia, polyuria, polyphagia, or weight loss. Which of the following laboratory reports confirms the diagnosis of diabetes?

a. One random glucose of 221 mg/dL
b. One random glucose reading of 221mg/dL, and another, on a later date, of 208 mg/dL
c. One fasting glucose measurement of 128 mg/dL
d. A glucose reading, taken 2 hours after a 75 g glucose load, of 163 mg/dL
e. A fasting glucose of 114 mg/dL, and a reading of 184 mg/dL 2 hours after a 75 g glucose load

424. An 18-year-old morbidly obese patient in your office is found to have a fasting glucose of 314 mg/dL. Which of the following test results indicates that he is a type 1 diabetic?

a. Low levels of c-peptide
b. Markedly elevated levels of c-peptide
c. Elevated levels of microalbumin in the urine
d. A markedly elevated hemoglobin A1C
e. Nerve conduction studies showing mild peripheral neuropathy

425. You are obtaining a family history from a new patient, and trying to determine her risk for various health conditions. She reports that her grandmother died of renal failure, but is unsure why her grandmother had that problem. What is the most common cause of end stage renal disease?

a. Hypertensive nephropathy
b. Diabetic nephropathy
c. Polycystic kidney disease
d. Glomerulonephritis
e. Contrast-induced nephropathy

426. You are managing a 36-year-old woman with a new diagnosis of type 2 diabetes. Her hemoglobin A1C was 7.2% at diagnosis. Her subsequent sugars were well-controlled using metformin, 1000 mg BID. At her visit 3 months later, her blood pressure is 100/72, her hemoglobin A1C was 6.0%, but her microalbumin screen is positive. Which of the following is the most appropriate response?

a. Continue weight loss and recheck in 3 months
b. Limit dietary protein intake
c. Intensify diabetic therapy to more tightly control glucose
d. Initiate therapy with an ACE inhibitor
e. Refer to nephrology

427. A 44-year-old man is seeing you for a routine diabetic check. He was diagnosed with type 2 diabetes 2 years ago. He is worried because his grandmother went blind as a complication from her diabetes. Which of the following statements about diabetic retinopathy is true?

a. The risk of retinopathy increases with increased hemoglobin A1C levels
b. It generally takes 10–20 years to see signs of retinopathy in a diabetic patient
c. A daily aspirin decreases the risk of retinopathy development
d. The first sign of retinopathy is usually the growth of new vessels on the retina
e. Retinopathy is an uncommon cause of visual loss in this day and age

428. You have just diagnosed a patient with type 2 diabetes. After discussing the importance of glucose control to limit long term complications from the illness, she asks what the most common cause of death is among diabetes. Which of the following is the answer to her question?

a. Heart disease
b. Pneumonia
c. Cancer
d. Stroke
e. Sepsis

429. You are seeing an African American man with newly diagnosed diabetes. His blood pressure at the last visit was 148/86, and at this visit it is 142/90. What should your first choice for blood pressure control be?

a. A beta-blocker
b. A thiazide diuretic
c. An ACE inhibitor
d. A calcium-channel blocker
e. An alpha-blocker

430. You are following a type 2 diabetic woman in her 50s. Six months ago, you checked her lipid profile. At that time, her total cholesterol was 245 mg/dL, her LDL was 148 mg/dL, her HDL was 30 mg/dL and her triglycerides were 362. She has tried lifestyle modifications, but despite losing weight and exercising, her profile hasn't substantially changed. What is the treatment of choice for this patient?

a. Continued lifestyle modifications
b. A 3-hydroxy-3-methylglutaryl coenzyme A (HMG-CoA) [P1]reductase inhibitor (a "statin")
c. Niacin
d. Fibric acid derivatives
e. A bile acid resin

431. A 39-year old diabetic man asks you questions about his diet. Which of the following is true?

a. A high fiber diet improves glycemic control
b. A low carbohydrate diet improves glycemic control
c. A high protein diet improves glycemic control
d. Sucrose should not be included in the diabetic diet
e. A formalized dietary program is more likely to produce long term sustained effects

432. A 44-year-old African American with type 2 diabetes transfers care to you. Reviewing her records, you find she is on the maximum dose of sulfonylurea, but her hemoglobin A1C is 9.2% (H). Review of her baseline laboratory tests reveals normal liver enzymes and a creatinine of 2.3 mg/dL. Which of the following management options would be most beneficial?

a. Change to another sulfonylurea
b. Add a biguanide
c. Add a meglitinide
d. Add a thiazolidinedione
e. Add an alpha-glucosidase inhibitor

433. A 48-year-old woman has been treated for type 2 diabetes for 6 years with metformin 2000 mg daily, and glyburide 10 mg daily. She is modestly compliant with her diet, medications, and exercise. She is 69 in. tall and weighs 278 lb. Her most recent HbA$_{1C}$ is 8.2% which has been relatively unchanged over the past 18 months. If weight loss is a therapeutic priority for this patient, which of the following would represent a logical next step?

a. Increase her glyburide to the maximum dose of 10 mg twice daily
b. Add a long-acting, basal insulin such as insulin glargine, discontinue glyburide, and maintain metformin
c. Add an insulin sensitizing agent such a pioglitazone or rosiglitazone to her regimen
d. Add an incretin-mimetic such as exenatide to her regimen
e. Simplify the regimen by discontinuing all oral medications and substituting a long-acting basal insulin plus a rapid-acting preprandial insulin such as insulin aspart

434. You have been treating a 46-year-old woman for type 2 diabetes for 2 years with metformin 2000 mg daily. She is compliant with her diet and medications, and exercises regularly. She is 65 in. tall and weighs 200 lb. Her most recent HbA$_{1C}$ is 8.0% which is elevated from 7.8% 3 months ago. You added the insulin-sensitizing agent rosiglitizone to her regimen 2 weeks ago. The patient presents today complaining of a problem that she attributes to the new medication. Which of the following is a likely complaint?

a. Symptomatic hypoglycemia
b. Edema and weight gain
c. Cough
d. Paradoxical hyperglycemia
e. Gastrointestinal intolerance

435. A 48-year-old man with type 2 diabetes talks to you at a routine appointment about a drug he heard discussed on the news. This patient currently takes gliplizide, pioglitazone, and acarbose. He wants to know more about sitagliptin (Januvia). Which of the following best explains its mechanism of action?

a. Inhibition of glucagon release
b. Increases the sensitivity of the body to insulin
c. Inhibition of hepatic gluconeogenesis
d. Inhibition of gastric emptying
e. Suppression of glucagon elaboration and delayed gastric emptying

436. You are thinking about starting a type 2 diabetic on insulin therapy to improve her glucose control. Which of the following insulin types has the most rapid onset of action?

a. Aspart (Novolog)
b. Regular
c. Lente
d. Ultralente
e. Glargine (Lantus)

437. You are thinking about starting a type 2 diabetic on insulin therapy to improve her glucose control. Which of the following insulin preparations has a peak or maximum action at approximately 5 hours?

a. Aspart (Novolog)
b. Regular
c. Lente
d. Ultralente
e. Glargine (Lantus)

438. You are thinking about starting a type 2 diabetic on insulin therapy to improve her glucose control. Which of the following insulin preparations has the longest duration of action?

a. Aspart (Novolog)
b. Regular
c. Lente
d. Ultralente
e. Glargine (Lantus)

439. After a period of noncompliance, one of your type 1 diabetics has been hospitalized for diabetic ketoacidosis. He has required approximately 100 units of insulin in a 24-hour period in the hospital using a sliding scale. You decide to begin split-dose therapy with neutral protamine Hagedorn (NPH) and regular insulin. How much NPH insulin should be given to this patient in the morning?

a. 25 units
b. 33 units
c. 50 units
d. 66 units
e. 75 units

440. You are caring for a type 1 diabetic who has been hospitalized with diabetic ketoacidosis, and determining an appropriate insulin regimen for her. She has required 60 units of insulin per day to maintain adequate control in the hospital. You decide to use insulin glargine (Lantus) and aspart (Lispro) in combination. What should her Lantus dose be?

a. 10 units
b. 20 units
c. 30 units
d. 40 units
e. 50 units

441. You have maximized oral therapy for a type 2 diabetic in your office. She works hard at diet and exercise, and is on maximal doses of oral hypoglycemics, but her glycosolated hemoglobin is 8.6%. You decide to add insulin to her regimen. She is currently 67 in tall and weighs 100 kg. How much neutral protamine Hagedorn (NPH) should you give her at night as an addition to her current regimen?

a. 5 units
b. 10 units
c. 15 units
d. 20 units
e. 25 units

442. A 62-year-old woman sees you for preoperative clearance for a right hip replacement. Her past medical history is significant for hypertension, chronic kidney disease, osteoarthritis and type 2 diabetes. During your examination, you detect a painless mass in her lower right abdomen. You schecule a CT scan with angiographic contrast. Which one of this patients' medications should be held prior to her receiving radiocontrast dye?

a. Metoprolol XL 100 mg
b. Metformin ER 1000 mg
c. Lisinopril 20 mg
d. Aspirin 325 mg
e. Pentoxifylline 400 mg

443. You are caring for a 28-year-old man with dyslipidemia. Specifically, he has hypoalphalipoproteinemia (low high-density lipoprotein). Which of the following interventions is more likely to raise his HDL levels?

a. Cigarette smoking
b. Alcohol in moderation
c. Weight loss
d. Low dietary intake of cholesterol
e. Stress reduction

444. You have performed a screening lipid profile on an otherwise healthy man. His results indicate elevated triglycerides, a low high-density lipoprotein, a high low-density lipoprotein, an elevated total cholesterol, and an elevated very low-density lipoprotein. You'd like to rescreen him in the fasting state. Which of the following laboratory values is likely to decrease in the fasting state?

a. Serum triglycerides
b. High-density lipoprotein
c. Low-density lipoprotein
d. Total cholesterol
e. Very low-density lipoprotein

445. You did screening cholesterol tests on a 33-year-old man and found his results to be:

> Total cholesterol: 220 mg/dL (H)
> Low-density lipoprotein: 125 mg/dL (H)
> High-density lipoprotein: 34 mg/dL (L)
> Triglycerides: 307 mg/dL (H)
> C-reactive protein: 2.4 mg/dL (H)

Which of his lab results is the best predictor of an adverse outcome in this patient?

a. Total cholesterol
b. Low-density lipoprotein
c. High-density lipoprotein
d. Triglycerides
e. C-reactive protein

446. In an effort to become more healthy overall, a 28-year-old woman with dyslipidemia decides to quit smoking. What effect would you expect this to have on her lipid profile?

a. Decrease total cholesterol
b. Decrease low-density lipoprotein
c. Decrease fasting triglycerides
d. Increase high-density lipoprotein
e. Decrease very low-density lipoprotein

447. You are prescribing niacin for a patient with elevated LDL and triglycerides. He complains of flushing with the medication. What is the best way for this patient to avoid flushing with this medication?

a. Take niacin at night
b. Take aspirin before taking niacin
c. Take niacin with food
d. Take niacin on an empty stomach
e. Take niacin with milk

448. You are beginning an HMG-CoA reductase inhibitor on a patient with elevated total cholesterol and a low high-density lipoprotein level. You are concerned about drug interactions with this class of medications. Which of the following medications is less likely to cause drug interactions?

a. Atorvastatin
b. Simvastatin
c. Lovastatin
d. Lovastatin-niacin
e. Pravastatin

449. In an attempt to lower cholesterol through diet, you recommend that a 40-year-old male take fish oil. What is the lipid lowering mechanism of action of fish oil?

a. Sequesters bile acids
b. Changes hepatic metabolism of lipoprotein
c. Inhibits HMG-CoA reductase
d. Interferes with cholesterol absorption in the gut
e. Decreases secretions of triglycerides by the liver

450. You are seeing a 28-year-old man with significantly elevated triglycerides. You are considering gemfibrozil (Lopid) therapy. What is the mechanism of action of gemfibrozil?

a. Sequesters bile acids
b. Changes hepatic metabolism of lipoprotein
c. Inhibits HMG-CoA reductase
d. Interferes with cholesterol absorption in the gut
e. Decreases secretions of triglycerides by the liver

451. You are working with a 44-year-old man with difficult to manage dyslipidemia. He is taking atorvastatin (Lipitor) at maximum dosages, and you are considering adding ezetemibe (Zetia) to improve the lipid profile. How does ezetemibe work to help lower cholesterol?

a. Sequestration of bile acids
b. Changing hepatic metabolism of lipoproteins
c. Inhibits HMG-CoA reductase
d. Interferes with cholesterol absorption in the gut
e. Decreases secretion of triglycerides by the liver

452. You are seeing a 26-year-old sexually active man who presents to obtain HIV testing. You perform appropriate pretest counseling and determine his risks to be low. He is heterosexual, has never had sex with prostitutes or a known HIV positive woman, his last sexual activity was more than 6 months ago, and he has never used IV drugs or had a transfusion. His test is negative. Which of the following is the best way to deliver the results?

a. Copy the results and send them to his home
b. Call him on his home telephone
c. Call him on his personal cell phone
d. Discuss the results in person during an office visit
e. Agree on the method at his pretest visit, and comply with the patient's wishes

453. You are taking care of a 22-year-old woman with fever, aches and fatigue. Her history reveals intravenous drug abuse, and you suspect acute HIV infection. Which of the following tests is best to rule out acute HIV?

a. Enzyme-linked immunosorbent assay (ELISA)
b. Western blot
c. Immunofluroescent antibody test
d. Quantitative plasma HIV RNA (viral load)
e. P24 antigen assay

454. You are caring for a patient newly diagnosed with HIV infection. Initial laboratory work revealed a positive Hepatitis B surface antibody, and a positive Hepatitis A antibody. His immunization history is unknown. Which of the following vaccines should be administered to this patient?

a. Hepatitis A
b. Hepatitis B
c. Pneumococcal vaccine
d. MMR vaccine
e. Oral polio vaccine

455. You are caring for a 38-year-old woman with a long history of intravenous drug abuse. She was diagnosed with HIV 2 years ago, and has been doing well on therapy without disease progression. You order a purified protein derivative skin test for TB. What amount of induration indicates a positive test?

a. Any induration indicates a positive test
b. 3 mm
c. 5 mm
d. 10 mm
e. 15 mm

456. One of your patients has failed therapy for HIV, and his CD4 lymphocyte counts are falling. During his last two visits, his CD4 count has been less than 50 lymphocytes/mm^3. Prophylaxis for which of the following should be instituted at this time?

a. *Mycobacterium avium* complex
b. Fungal infections
c. Herpes simplex
d. Herpes zoster
e. Cytomegalovirus

457. You are seeing a patient with a long-standing HIV infection. The patient has been unable to afford his medication regimen and has been off medication for several months. He presents with shortness of breath. Blood gasses obtained emergently reveal a PaO_2 of 65 mm Hg. His chest x-ray is shown below:

(Reproduced, with permission, from Knoop K, Stack L, Storrow A. Atlas of Emergency Medicine, 2nd ed. New York: McGraw-Hill, 2002: 666.)

Assuming the patient is not allergic, which of the following is the best first-line treatment?

a. Azithromycin
b. Trimethoprim-sulfamethoxazole
c. Trimethoprim-sulfamethoxazole and corticosteroids
d. Triple drug treatment against tuberculosis
e. Quadruple drug treatment against tuberculosis

458. You have seen a 36-year-old man with elevated blood pressure. On one occasion, his blood pressure was 163/90 mm Hg, and on a second occasion, his blood pressure was 158/102 mm Hg. You have encouraged lifestyle modifications including weight loss using exercise and dietary changes. Despite some modest weight loss, at his current visit, his blood pressure is 166/92 mm Hg. Which of the following is the best treatment strategy at this point?

a. Use a thiazide diuretic
b. Use an ACE inhibitor

c. Use an angiotensin receptor blocker
d. Use a beta-blocker
e. Use a two drug combination of medications

459. You are examining a 40-year-old patient for the first time, and find her blood pressure to be 155/92 mm Hg. Which of the following physical examination findings, if present, would indicate a secondary cause of hypertension?

a. A left-sided carotid bruit
b. Distended jugular veins
c. A precordial heave
d. Absence of a femoral pulse
e. Papilledema

460. You have just diagnosed a 35-year-old man with hypertension. He is otherwise healthy and has no complaints. Which of the following laboratory tests is *not* indicated in the initial workup?

a. Hemoglobin and hematocrit
b. Potassium
c. A thyroid stimulating hormone level
d. Fasting glucose
e. A resting electrocardiogram

461. You are treating a 40-year-old man for hypertension. He is not responding well to a thiazide diuretic, and on further evaluation reports intermittent tachycardia, diaphoresis, and dizziness upon standing. Which of the following tests is most likely to help you evaluate these symptoms?

a. Chest x-ray
b. Captopril renal scan
c. Urinary metanephrines and vanillymandelic acid levels
d. Plasma renin activity levels
e. Echocardiogram

462. You are treating a 61-year-old man for hypertension. He is not responding well to combination therapy with a thiazide diuretic and a beta-blocker. On physical examination, you note an abdominal bruit. Which of the following tests is most likely to help you evaluate him further?

a. Chest x-ray
b. Captopril renal scan
c. Urinary metanephrines and vanillymandelic acid levels
d. Aortic CT scan
e. Echocardiogram

463. You are counseling a 33-year-old obese woman with hypertension. Which of the following interventions would lower her systolic blood pressure the most?

a. Weight loss amounting to 10% of her total body weight
b. Adopting a diet high in fruits, vegetables, and low fat dairy products
c. Restricting dietary sodium
d. Increasing physical activity at least 30 minutes a day, most days of the week
e. Limit alcohol consumption to no more than 1 drink per day

464. Despite lifestyle changes, a 37-year-old patient of yours still has blood pressures above goal. She has no other medical concerns, and no abnormalities on physical examination or initial laboratory evaluation. Which of the following medications is best as an initial first line monotherapy?

a. A thiazide diuretic
b. An ACE inhibitor
c. An angiotensin receptor blocker
d. A calcium-channel blocker
e. A beta-blocker

465. A 42-year-old male patient of yours presented to the emergency department with a stroke. After full recovery, he presents to your office for follow up. Assuming he has no other medical concerns, which of the following medications is best to lower his blood pressure and prevent recurrent stroke?

a. An aldosterone antagonist
b. An ACE inhibitor
c. An angiotensin receptor blocker
d. A calcium-channel blocker
e. A beta-blocker

466. A 55-year-old man comes to your office after not being seen by a physician in more than 10 years. He is found to be hypertensive, and his creatinine is found to be 2.3 mg/dL (H). Which medication is likely to be best to control his blood pressure and decrease the likelihood of progression of his renal disease?

a. A thiazide diuretic
b. An ACE inhibitor
c. A calcium-channel blocker
d. A beta-blocker
e. An aldosterone antagonist

467. You have diagnosed a 39-year-old woman with hypertension. Lifestyle modifications helped reduce her blood pressure, but she was still above goal.

You chose to start hydrochlorothiazide, 25 mg daily. This helped her blood pressure, but her blood pressure is still 142/94. Which of the following is the best approach to take in this situation?

a. Increase her hydrochlorothiazide to 50 mg per day
b. Change to a loop diuretic
c. Change to an ACE inhibitor
d. Change to a beta-blocker
e. Add an ACE inhibitor

468. You are seeing a 49-year-old man with a known history of hypercholesterolemia and hypertension who has had recent complaints of chest pain. He reports a chest pressure, described as "heaviness" in the substernal area. It is not associated with activity, but will occur intermittently throughout the day. Which of the following is the best way to describe what the patient is feeling?

a. Classic angina
b. Atypical angina
c. Anginal equivalent
d. Nonanginal pain
e. Atypical nonanginal pain

469. You are seeing a 36-year-old man complaining of shortness of breath. He reports symptoms associated with activity and relieved by rest. He is otherwise healthy, takes no medications, and denies chest pain or pressure. Which of the following is the best way to describe what the patient is feeling?

a. Classic angina
b. Atypical angina
c. Anginal equivalent
d. Nonanginal pain
e. Atypical nonanginal pain

470. You are seeing a 44-year-old woman with a known history of asthma who has had recent complaints of chest pain. She reports a stabbing pain that seems to be worse with inspiration. It is not associated with activity, but will occur intermittently throughout the day. Which of the following is the best way to describe what the patient is feeling?

a. Classic angina
b. Atypical angina
c. Anginal equivalent
d. Nonanginal pain
e. Atypical nonanginal pain

471. You are evaluating a 39-year-old otherwise healthy man with a family history of ischemic heart disease. He describes chest pressure that radiates to his jaw when he walks up steps at work. You order an ECG in the office, shown below:

(Reproduced, with permission, from Ferry D. Basic Electrocardiography in Ten Days, 1st ed. New York: McGraw-Hill, 2001: 83.)

What is the test of choice to determine if his chest pain is due to cardiac ischemia?

a. Exercise treadmill test
b. Thallium exercise treadmill test
c. Stress echocardiogram
d. Persantine/thallium test
e. Dobutamine echocardiogram

472. You are caring for a 56-year-old man who presents to you for an evaluation of chest pain. You determine that an exercise treadmill test is necessary. The patient completes stage III of a Bruce protocol, achieves a heart rate of 136 beats per minute, and has an ST segment depression of 1 mm in the three inferior leads at a heart rate of 130 beats per minute. These changes lasted 2 minutes into recovery. Which of the following features is a poor prognostic sign for the patient?

a. Being unable to reach stage IV of a Bruce protocol
b. Failure to achieve a heart rate of 140 beats per minute
c. Onset of ST segment depression at a heart rate of 130 beats per minute
d. Having ST segment depression in multiple leads
e. Having ST segment depression lasting two minutes into recovery

473. You are medically treating an 85-year-old woman with stable angina, and choose to use nitrates. What is the most important consideration when using this medication?

a. Headache
b. Fatigue
c. Interactions with beta-blockers
d. Interactions with calcium-channel blockers
e. Development of tolerance

474. You have chosen to treat a 70-year-old man with ischemic heart disease using a beta-blocker. What is the most appropriate endpoint for the use of beta-blockers in this case?

a. Use no more than the equivalent of 40 mg BID of propalolol
b. Use the amount necessary to achieve a blood pressure of 100/70 mmHg or less
c. Use the amount necessary to keep the heart rate between 50–60 beats per minute
d. Increase the dosage until fatigue limits use
e. Increase the amount until angina disappears

475. You are seeing a 25-year-old man for a complete physical examination. Evaluating his height and weight, you determine his body mass index (BMI) to be 32. How would you classify this patient?

a. His BMI classifies him as being underweight
b. His BMI places him within the normal range
c. His BMI classifies him as being overweight
d. His BMI classifies him as obese
e. His BMI classifies him as morbidly obese

476. A 33-year-old woman is seeing you for weight management. At 5 ft 6in tall and 230 lb, she reports a history of having difficulty with weight since her teenage years. She has tried several "fad" diets but seems to gain weight quickly when going off the diet. She takes oral contraceptives to "help regulate her period," but the rest of her medical history is unremarkable. Her vital signs are within the normal range. On physical examination, she has moderate adult acne and mild facial hair growth. The rest of her examination is unremarkable. Which of the following is the most likely secondary cause contributing to her obesity?

a. Polycystic ovary syndrome
b. Cushing syndrome
c. Hypogonadism
d. Hypothyroidism
e. Hypopituitary syndrome

477. You are discussing weight management with an obese 33-year-old male patient. In an effort to help motivate him to lose weight, you choose to bring up some health complications of obesity. Obesity increases the risk of developing which of the following diseases?

a. Hypothyroidism
b. Arthritis
c. Cushing's disease
d. Asthma
e. Osteoporosis

478. You are working with a 48-year-old type 2 diabetic, diagnosed 1 month ago. The patient wishes to lose weight to help manage his illness, but is not really interested in exercise. You work with him on a dietary plan that diminishes his daily calorie intake by 500 calories per day. All things being equal, how much weight can this patient expect to lose in 6 weeks?

a. 3 lb
b. 6 lb
c. 9 lb
d. 12 lb
e. 15 lb

479. After 2 months of working on diet and attempting an exercise program, a patient complains of making limited progress. Indeed, her weight has stayed stable despite engaging in 20 minutes of walking 3 days per week, and limiting caloric intake. She asks if she can try medication to help with her weight loss goals. Which of the following is true regarding the use of medication in weight loss programs?

a. Medications used for weight loss are unsafe and should be avoided
b. There is no role for medications in weight loss programs
c. Short courses of some medications have been shown to be helpful in initiating and maintaining weight loss
d. Long courses of some medications have been shown to be helpful in initiating and maintaining weight loss
e. Medications can be a helpful adjunct to a weight loss program

480. A 49-year-old African American perimenopausal woman is seeing you after having fractured her wrist. Her past medical history is significant for oral contraceptive use for 20 years, obesity and Grave's disease leading to current hypothyroidism. She nursed two children for 6 months each. Which component of the patient's history puts her at increased risk for osteoporosis?

a. African American race
b. Oral contraceptive use
c. Obesity
d. Grave's disease
e. Breast feeding

481. A 32-year-old woman is seeing you because her mother has been diagnosed with osteoporosis. She asks you what type of exercise will help her prevent the development of the disease. According to recommendations, which of the following exercises is recommended to help maintain bone mass?

a. Tennis
b. Swimming
c. Cycling
d. Skating
e. Skiing

482. You are caring for a 48-year-old Caucasian woman with a history of anorexia nervosa in her late 20s. She was an elite track and field athlete in her late teens and early 20s, and was considered for the US Olympic team in her prime. Which of the following options is best for primary osteoporosis screening in this woman?

a. History
b. Physical examination
c. Serum calcium
d. Serum human osteocalcin levels
e. Bone density imaging

483. You are evaluating a 76-year-old woman on long-term glucocortico-steroid therapy for polymyalgia rheumatica. Which of the following is the diagnostic imaging test of choice to diagnose osteoporosis?

a. Plain radiographs
b. Single photon absorptiometry
c. Dual photon absorptiometry
d. Dual energy x-ray absorptiometry
e. Quantitative computerized tomography of bone

484. You screened a 52-year-old, at-risk woman for osteoporosis using a DEXA scan. You received a T-score and a Z-score in the report. Which of the following indicates osteoporosis?

a. An equal T- and Z-score
b. A T-score of +2.5
c. A T-score of −2.5
d. A Z-score of +2.5
e. A Z-score of −2.5

485. You have diagnosed a 53-year-old woman with osteoporosis. She is postmenopausal, and you are considering estrogen replacement therapy. Which of the following is *not* an absolute contraindication to estrogen replacement therapy?

a, A history of breast cancer
b. A history of uterine cancer
c. A history of estrogen-dependent neoplasia
d. Abnormal genital bleeding
e. A history of a thromboembolic disorder

486. You are treating an elderly postmenopausal woman with osteoporosis. She recently suffered an acute osteoporotic vertebral fracture, and is suffering from secondary pain. Which osteoporosis treatment also has analgesic effects with respect to bone pain?

a. Estrogen
b. The combination of calcium and vitamin D
c. Calcitonin
d. Alendronate (Fosamax)
e. Raloxifene (Evista)

487. You have just diagnosed osteoporosis in a postmenopausal woman. She is considering treatment alternatives and wonders about the bisphosphonates. Which of the following is the best description of how this class of medications works?

a. They increase calcium absorption in the gastrointestinal (GI) tract
b. They block the activity of the cytokines that stimulate bone reabsorption
c. They bind to bone surfaces to inhibit osteoclast activity
d. They stimulate osteoblasts and increase bone formation
e. They mimic estrogen's effect on bone

488. You are seeing a 32-year-old woman for fatigue. Your differential diagnosis includes major depressive disorder, but she does not describe a depressed or irritable mood. Of the following choices, which symptom of depression must be present in order to diagnose a major depressive disorder in someone without depressed mood?

a. Sleep changes
b. Loss of interest or pleasure in usually enjoyable activities
c. Guilt or feelings of worthlessness
d. Loss of energy
e. Change in appetite

489. You have just diagnosed depression in an otherwise healthy adult male. He has agreed to start an antidepressant medication, but is concerned about sexual side effects. Which of the following medications is least likely to cause sexual side effects in this patient?

a. Bupropion
b. Citalopram
c. Fluoxetine
d. Sertraline
e. Venlafaxine

490. You are discussing treatment options for a 43-year-old woman with major depressive disorder. Which of the following is a true statement regarding the effectiveness of treatment for depressive disorders?

a. Only about 25% of patients that receive medication alone will find the medication to be effective
b. Patients who find one medication ineffective are likely to find all medications ineffective
c. In order to prevent a relapse of depressive symptoms, patients should continue treatment for 3–4 months
d. In general, patients respond best to the combination of medication and counseling
e. Electroconvulsive therapy is ineffective when compared with newer medical therapy

491. You are treating a 48-year-old man for major depression. His medical history includes a head injury several years ago that has left him with a seizure disorder. Which of the following antidepressants would be contraindicated?

a. Venlafaxine
b. Nefazodone
c. Mirtazapine
d. Fluoxetine
e. Bupropion

492. Which of the following conditions is considered an anxiety disorder?

a. Social phobia
b. Conversion disorder
c. Somatization disorder
d. Anorexia nervosa
e. Histrionic personality disorder

493. You are following a 16-year-old girl with a suspected eating disorder. Which of the following, if present, would help differentiate anorexia nervosa from bulimia nervosa?

a. Binge eating or purging
b. The use of laxatives, diuretics, or enemas
c. Self-evaluation is unduly influenced by body weight and shape
d. Episodic lack of control over eating
e. Inappropriate behaviors to prevent weight gain

494. Which of the following is a major risk factor for the development of attention-deficit/hyperactivity disorder (ADHD)?

a. Environmental exposure to tobacco smoke
b. Environmental allergies
c. A family history of ADHD
d. Low self-esteem
e. Academic underachievement

495. A 26-year-old male college graduate is seeing you for an office visit. He is concerned that he may have adult ADHD. Which of the following is true regarding this condition?

a. The symptoms are likely to be more pronounced in adults as compared with children
b. Children diagnosed with ADHD commonly continue to have symptoms into adulthood

c. Sleep disturbance is a distinctive feature of adult ADHD
d. Appetite disturbance is a distinctive feature of adult ADHD
e. The symptom picture of adult ADHD mimics that in children

496. What is the principal mechanism by which stimulant medications work to improve symptoms of ADHD?

a. Inhibition of serotonin reuptake
b. Stimulation of serotonin production
c. Inhibition of dopamine and norepinephrine reuptake
d. Stimulation of dopamine and norepinepherine production
e. Blocking the release of serotonin

497. A 45-year-old woman presents to your office for evaluation. She reports that over the last few weeks, she's noted an enlarging mass in the front of her neck. She feels well, has had no changes in her health, and denies symptoms of hyper- or hypothyroidism. She also denies recent viral illness. On examination, you note a diffusely enlarged thyroid that is tender to touch. What is her most likely diagnosis?

a. Hashimoto's thyroiditis
b. Subacute lymphocytic thyroiditis
c. Subacute granulomatous thyroiditis
d. Suppurative thyroiditis
e. Invasive fibrous thyroiditis

498. A 26-year-old woman presents with weight gain, lethargy, dry skin, sweatiness, cold intolerance, and thinning hair. You suspect hypothyroidism and order the appropriate laboratory tests. Her thyroid stimulating hormone is high, and her free T3 and free T4 are both low. Which of the following is the most likely diagnosis?

a. Primary hypothyroidism
b. Secondary hypothyroidism
c. Iodine deficiency
d. Thyroid hormone resistance
e. Subclinical hypothyroidism

499. You are screening a 35-year-old woman who presents with tachycardia, nervousness, tremor, palpitations, heat intolerance, and weight loss. You suspect Graves' disease. What single test is best for differentiating Graves' disease from other causes of hyperthyroidism?

a. Thyroid stimulating hormone
b. TSH with free T4 and free T3
c. Thyroid receptor antibodies
d. Radionucleotide imaging of the thyroid
e. Thyroid ultrasound

500. When examining a 35-year-old, you notice a firm 3 cm thyroid nodule. His thyroid studies are normal, and he is clinically euthyroid. Radionucleotide imaging demonstrates uptake in the thyroid nodule. What is the most likely diagnosis?

a. Colloid cyst
b. Thyroid adenoma
c. Thyroid carcinoma
d. Metastatic disease
e. Neurofibroma

Chronic Conditions

Answers

338. The answer is c. (*South-Paul, pp 221–230.*) The sexual response is divided into four phases. The first is libido (or desire/interest). This phase requires androgens and an intact sensory system. In men, this is more visual-based, but in women it is more relationship-based. The second phase is arousal (or excitement) and in men, involves erection. This requires an intact parasympathetic nervous system and vascular system. The next phase is orgasm, and in men involves ejaculation. This phase requires an intact sympathetic system.

339. The answer is b. (*South-Paul, pp 221–230.*) In patients with decreased sex drive, laboratory workup should be directed by the history and physical examination findings. In a patient with no other complaints and no physical examination findings, assessment of hormone status is indicated. Testosterone levels should be checked in the morning, when they peak. Free testosterone is a more accurate measure of androgen status, as it is a measure of bioavailable testosterone. The TSH and prolactin levels may be indicated in the presence of other complaints or physical findings. PSA would not be helpful.

340. The answer is c. (*South-Paul, pp 221–230.*) Many medications can cause sexual dysfunction. Medications that commonly cause ejaculatory dysfunction in men include beta-blockers, alpha-blockers, antipsychotics and selective serotonin reuptake inhibitors. Hydrochlorozide can cause erectile dysfunction and decreased libido. Omeprazole and bupropion often do not negatively impact sexual functioning.

341. The answer is e. (*South-Paul, pp 221–230.*) Tricyclics and selective serotonin reuptake inhibitors frequently cause sexual dysfunction. Bupropion actually decreases the orgasm threshold and is least likely to cause sexual dysfunction.

342. The answer is b. (*South-Paul, pp 221–230.*) Premature ejaculation is the most common sexual dysfunction in men, affecting about 29% of the general population. Alprostadil is used for erectile dysfunction, but would not positively effect premature ejaculation. Fluoxetine raises the threshold for orgasm, making it an effective treatment option. Bupropion and silendafil may decrease the orgasmic threshold and might be problematic. Atenolol may cause erectile dysfunction, but would likely not treat premature ejaculation.

343. The answer is b. (*Mengel, pp 593–603.*) Characteristics known to influence the epidemiology of substance use disorders include gender (men are more likely to be affected than women), age (disorders become less frequent with age), marital status (single persons have a higher risk than married), employment (the unemployed are at higher risk), and level of education (less educated persons are at higher risk). Though one would expect job stress to influence substance use, studies have not shown this to be true.

344. The answer is c. (*Mengel, pp 593–603.*) Most clinicians agree that psychiatric disorders cannot be reliably assessed in patients who are currently or recently intoxicated. Alcohol is a depressant, and may be the main factor in the patient's depressed symptoms. Detoxification and a period of abstinence is necessary before an evaluation for other psychiatric disorders can be effectively completed.

345. The answer is d. (*Mengel, pp 593–603.*) Most people that abuse alcohol likely have completely normal laboratory studies. However, of the tests listed in the question, the GGT is the most sensitive. Elevated GGT is shown to be more sensitive than an elevated MCV, ALT, AST, or LDH. The specificity of the GGT is low, however, being elevated in nonalcoholic liver disease, diabetes, pancreatitis, hyperthyroidism, heart failure, and anticonvulsant use.

346. The answer is b. (*Mengel, pp 593–603.*) Drugs used for addiction work in one of four ways. They either cause the body to have a negative reaction to an ingested drug, reduce the reinforcing effects of an ingested drug, block the effects of the drug by binding to the receptor site, or saturate the receptor sites with agonists that do not create the drug's desired effect. Naltrexone is known to be helpful for both opiate addiction and alcohol addiction. Naltrexone saturates opiate receptor sites and leaves them unavailable for opiate attachment. For alcohol abuse, naltrexone works differently, reducing the reinforcing effect of alcohol (not allowing patients to become "drunk").

347. The answer is a. (*Mengel, pp 593–603.*) Disulfiram cause the body to have a negative reaction to ingested alcohol, regardless of the form. As such, it is a deterrent. The reaction to alcohol that occurs is manifested by flushing, nausea, and vomiting. Importantly, alcohol in cough medicines, mouthwashes, and other forms must be avoided, as the reaction does not discriminate based on from where the alcohol comes.

348. The answer is b. (*Rakel, pp 1339–1345.*) The nicotine withdrawal syndrome is a serious obstacle for patients wishing to stop smoking. Withdrawal symptoms often begin within hours after the last cigarette. Early abstinence is characterized by irritability, anxiety, restlessness, depressed mood, inattention, and insomnia. Nicotine replacement is often effective in lessening some of these symptoms, as is bupropion.

349. The answer is d. (*Rakel, pp 1339–1345.*) Nicotine nasal spray offers the fastest delivery of nicotine. This is followed by gum (if used correctly), lozenges, and inhalation. The nicotine patch releases nicotine the most slowly and gradually.

350. The answer is c. (*Rakel, pp 1339–1345.*) Cocaine withdrawal does not produce a significant physiologic withdrawal. Intoxication with cocaine does produce elevated heart rate and blood pressure. The most common problem produced by cocaine withdrawal is known as a "crash." The crash is characterized by extreme fatigue and significant depression. Relapse is common during the crash because return to use provides quick and reliable relief.

351. The answer is c. (*Rakel, pp 1339–1345.*) Opiate withdrawal is well-characterized, and although not life-threatening in otherwise healthy adults, can cause severe discomfort. Symptoms from a short-acting drug like heroin can occur within just a few hours. Withdrawal from longer acting opiates may not cause symptoms for days. Early symptoms include lacrimation, rhinorrhea, yawning, and diaphoresis. Restlessness and irritability occur later, with bone pain, nausea, diarrhea, abdominal cramping, and mood lability occurring even later.

Cocaine does not have a significant physiologic withdrawal syndrome, but craving is intense. Marijuana withdrawal syndrome is also not physiologically significant. Ecstasy can be considered a hallucinogen or a stimulant, and withdrawal is often associated with depression, but not the symptoms described above. Benzodiazepine withdrawal mimics alcohol withdrawal, and is associated with hypertension, tachycardia, and possibly seizures.

352. The answer is a. (*South-Paul, pp 265–284.*) The picture shown demonstrates Heberden's nodes (at the distal interphalangeal joints) and Bouchard's nodes (at the proximal interphalangeal joints). These abnormalities are commonly classified as osteoarthritis, but are only infrequently associated with pain or disability. Laboratory evaluation will only rarely show an inflammatory process, and an elevated uric acid level would be an incidental finding.

353. The answer is b. (*South-Paul, pp 265–284.*) Osteoarthritis is characterized as being pauciarticular. The pain is worse with activity and improved with rest. There is often mild swelling, but warmth and an effusion are rare. Crepitus is common, as is malalignment of the joint. Rheumatoid arthritis tends to be polyarticular and symmetric. Morning stiffness improves with activity. Gout is abrupt in onset and monoarticular. Tendonitis and fibromyalgia are not associated with joint swelling and crepitus.

354. The answer is c. (*South-Paul, pp 265–284.*) The patient's history is consistent with an attack of gout. The most common presentation of gout is podagra (an abrupt, intense inflammation of the first MTP joint), but any joint can be affected. It is characterized by an abrupt onset of monoarticular symptoms with pain at rest and with movement. The attacks often occur overnight, after an inciting event (excessive alcohol or a heavy meal). The sufferer often cites exquisite pain, with even slight pressure on the joint being quite painful. Osteoarthritis and rheumatoid arthritis would not occur so abruptly. A stress fracture would likely not be as painful at rest, and cellulitis would generally not be as abrupt or painful.

Septic arthritis and gout may be clinically indistinguishable, unless the joint fluid is analyzed.

355. The answer is a. (*South-Paul, pp 265–284.*) Rheumatoid arthritis is characterized by gradual, symmetric involvement of joints, with morning stiffness. Hands and feet are usually involved first, but it may spread to larger joints. Fatigue is a common complaint. On examination, symmetric swelling and tenderness are common, with associated rheumatoid nodules. Osteoarthritis is generally less symmetric and often occurs later in life. Gout is usually monoarticular. Tendonitis and fibromyalgia would be less likely to be associated with joint swelling.

356. The answer is e. (*South-Paul, pp 265–284.*) Oral steroids have a strong potential for ulcer formation, and although they may offer temporary relief, would not be indicated for chronic osteoarthritis. Another steroid injection would be of limited benefit, and most recommend no more than two injections per year to avoid hastening of the osteoarthritic process. Ketorolac is not indicated for intra-articular injection. Hyaluronic acid injections have been shown to provide symptomatic relief in osteoarthritis for up to 6 months, but given the malalignment demonstrated in his x-ray, knee replacement would likely be more beneficial. Indications for replacement include poorly controlled pain despite maximal therapy, malalignment and decreased mobility or ambulation.

357. The answer is c. (*South-Paul, pp 265–284.*) Alcohol alters renal excretion of uric acid, allowing buildup of serum uric acid levels. This buildup allows crystals to precipitate in the joint spaces, causing the symptoms of gout.

358. The answer is d. (*South-Paul, pp 265–284.*) An evaluation of the joint aspirate is strongly recommended to establish the diagnosis of gout. It is critical to differentiate gout from infectious arthritis which is a medical emergency, and a joint aspirate will do this rapidly and accurately. The sedimentation rates and c-reactive protein are both nonspecific. Serum uric acid levels can be normal or high in the setting of acute gout. A 24-hour urine collection may help determine the most effective treatment for gout, but is not needed for diagnosis.

359. The answer is b. (*South-Paul, pp 265–284.*) The crystals typical of gout are needle-shaped and have negative birefringement. The crystals of pseudogout are rhomboid-shaped and demonstrate positive birefringement. Infectious arthritis, osteoarthritis and rheumatoid arthritis would not present with crystals in the joint aspirate.

360. The answer is c. (*South-Paul, pp 265–284.*) Infectious arthritis, gout and pseudogout may all be associated with cloudy joint aspirate fluid. The aspirate fluid obtained from a gout or pseudogout flare may also have a white blood cell count of 50,000 with a high proportion of polymorphonuclear leukocytes. However, glucose levels fluid aspirated from a knee with gout or pseudogout would be normal.

361. The answer is d. (*South-Paul, pp 265–284.*) Fluid aspirated from an osteoarthritic knee is characterized by generally clear joint fluid with a white blood cell count of 2–10,000. The distinguishing factor is the polymorphonuclear leukocytes. In rheumatoid arthritis, more than 50% of the WBCs are PMNs, while in osteoarthritis, less than 50% of the WBCs are PMNs.

362. The answer is a. *(South-Paul, pp 265–284.)* While a short course of nonsteroidal anti-inflammatory medication is one standard therapy for gout, another is a course of colchicine. Colchicine is given orally, one tablet every 1–2 hours until pain is controlled or side effects limit its use (the usual side effect is diarrhea). Most attacks respond to the first two or three pills, and the maximum number used in a 24 hour period is 6. Corticosteroids can provide quick relief, but should be reserved if initial therapy fails. Opiates may control pain, but will not lead to resolution of the inflammation. Allopurinol and probenecid are effective treatments for prevention, but should be used cautiously, as they can precpitiate a flare.

363. The answer is d. *(South-Paul, pp 265–284.)* Swelling of the proximal interphalangeal joints (shown here in the second and third fingers) is typical of rheumatoid arthritis. Symmetrical swelling is almost unique to rheumatoid arthritis, and even lupus, often confused with RA in the early stages, is rarely as consistently symmetrical. Fatigue is often out of proportion to the lack of sleep, and the prolonged morning stiffness in the history is essential to diagnosis.

364. The answer is a. *(South-Paul, pp 265–284.)* Extra-articular manifestations of RA can be seen at any stage of the disease. Most common are rheumatoid nodules that can occur anywhere on the body, but usually subcutaneously along pressure points. Vasculitis, dry eyes, dyspnea, or cough can all be seen. Cough and dyspnea may signal respiratory interstitial disease. Cardiac, GI, and renal systems are rarely involved. When a neuropathy is present, it is generally because of a compression syndrome, not as an extra-articular manifestation of the disease.

365. The answer is e. *(South-Paul, pp 265–284.)* In the past, most people treated the symptoms of RA with nonsteroidals until that was ineffective, then referred to rheumatology. Unfortunately, these agents did nothing to slow the progression of disease. The most important advancement in the treatment of rheumatoid arthritis has been the introduction of disease-modifying antirheumatic drugs (DMARDs). These agents not only control patient symptoms but suppress the underlying factors that result in synovitis, tissue reactivity, erosions, subluxations, and other complications. These should be managed by rheumatologists and started early to avoid or delay joint deformity.

366. The answer is d. (*Rakel, pp 918–924.*) Propranolol is a nonselective beta-blocker. They are contraindicated in asthma because they can trigger severe bronchospasm. The other choices would be appropriate in the right circumstances.

367. The answer is b. (*Rakel, pp 918–924.*) Environmental measures can be an important component of asthma control. They include keeping humidity in the home relatively low, under 50%, enclosing the mattress, box spring and pillows with allergen impermeable covers (they can be dust reservoirs), laundering bed linens with hot water, and removing carpeting whenever possible. Air filters have not been shown to affect reservoir levels of house dust mite allergens.

368. The answer is a. (*Mengel, pp 415–423.*) The most important component in the diagnosis of asthma is history. Patients with asthma typically have recurrent episodes of wheezing, but not all asthma includes wheezing, and not all wheezing is asthma. Cough is the only symptom in cough-variant asthma. Allergy testing may help to identify specific allergens, but is not useful in diagnosing asthma. A chest x-ray is useful to rule-out other causes of cough or wheezing, but is not needed to diagnose asthma. Pulmonary function testing is usually confirmatory, not diagnostic. Provocative testing is indicated for the rare patient in whom the diagnosis is in question, but should be used cautiously, as life-threatening bronchospasm may occur.

369. The answer is c. (*South-Paul, pp 308–327.*) Asthma is classified by its severity, assessing daytime and nighttime symptoms. Patients with symptoms less than twice a week, with brief exacerbations, and with nighttime symptoms less than twice a month are classified as having "mild intermittent" asthma. There is no "moderate intermittent" classification. The "mild persistent" classification refers to symptoms more than twice a week but less than once a day, with symptoms that sometimes affect usual activity. Nighttime symptoms occur more than twice a month. The "moderate persistent" classification is characterized by daily symptoms and use of short-acting inhaler, with exacerbations that affect activity and may last for days. Nighttime symptoms occur at least weekly. "Severe persistent" asthma is characterized by continual symptoms that limit physical activities, with frequent exacerbations and nighttime symptoms.

370. The answer is d. (*South-Paul, pp 308–327.*) The patient described in this question fits the "moderate persistent" classification, characterized by daily symptoms and use of short-acting inhaler, with exacerbations that affect activity and may last for days. Nighttime symptoms occur at least weekly.

371. The answer is c. (*South-Paul, pp 308–327. Mengel, pp 415–423.*) Peak flow measurements parallel the forced expiratory volume in 1 second (FEV_1), and are an easy and inexpensive way to monitor asthma control. The peak flow "zone system" allows patients' to monitor their control and participate in the clinical decision-making around their illness. Measurements between 80–100% of the patient's personal best are in the "green zone," and indicate that the patient is doing well. Measurements between 50–80% of the personal best are in the "yellow zone," and are a warning to consider a step up in therapy (review of medication technique, adherence, and environmental control, or use additional medication). Measurements below 50% of the personal best are an indicator that the patient needs immediate medical attention.

372. The answer is c. (*Rakel, pp 918–924.*) Inhaled corticosteroids are the mainstay of long-term asthma treatment, and act at numerous sites in the inflammatory cascade. They should be prescribed for all patients with all but very mild asthma. Changing short-acting agents would not likely be beneficial. Long-acting beta-agonists do not impact airway inflammation and should not be used without a corticosteroid. A leukotriene receptor antagonist is an option, but is generally thought of as a "second best" choice. Inhaled corticosteroids and leukotriene antagonists have replaced cromolyn in current asthma therapy.

373. The answer is b. (*Rakel, pp 918–924.*) The patient described in this question has worsening asthma symptoms and needs additional therapy. Long-acting beta-agonists are considered the most appropriate medication in this case, and are often packaged with an inhaled corticosteroid for ease of use. A leukotriene receptor antagonist would also be appropriate. A burst and taper of oral steroids may be appropriate for an acute flare, but not in this case. Cromolyn has associated compliance issues as it is dosed four times a day. Atrovent is usually not used unless there is a component of COPD, and theophylline, though an appropriate "third line" agent, is not more effective than a long-acting beta agonist.

374. The answer is b. (*Rakel, pp 918–924.*) Long-acting beta-agonists are less effective if not paired with inhaled corticosteroids. A leukotriene receptor antagonist is a better choice in this case. Cromolyn therapy has been replaced by newer agents, mainly because of compliance issues. Theophylline and oral steroids would not be indicated in this case.

375. The answer is a. (*Mengel, pp 273–277.*) Spondylolisthesis is the most common cause of low back pain in patients younger than age 26, especially athletes. Back strain is also a common diagnosis, but would generally follow an inciting event, and pain would be associated with movement. The patient is likely too young for osteoarthritis to be a consideration, and a lumbar disk herniation can occur at any age, but is less likely to be the diagnosis in this case. Neoplasm is a rare cause of low back pain.

376. The answer is d. (*Mengel, pp 273–277.*) Scoliosis is a common finding, especially in young females. The initial evaluation of an adolescent found to have scoliosis should focus on the severity of the curvature noted on x-ray. Adolescents with curvatures of less than 20° and no evidence of an underlying etiology can safely be followed with x-rays every 6 months to evaluate progression. Those with angles greater than 20° should be referred to an orthopedic specialist. Bracing has been shown to halt the progression of less severe curves, but would not be indicated unless progression is observed. Since 90% of thoracic curves are to the right, a left thoracic curve should be evaluated with an MRI.

377. The answer is b. (*Mengel, pp 273–277.*) Back pain caused by an inflammatory condition (rheumatoid arthritis, ankylosing spondylitis, Reiter's syndrome) are rare, but have characteristics that are helpful in differentiating them from other causes of pain. Inflammatory conditions generally produce greater pain and stiffness in the morning, while mechanical disorders tend to worsen throughout the day with activity. A disk herniation might be associated with radiation and neurological symptoms. A compression fracture would begin suddenly, and a neoplasm is unlikely to get better throughout the day.

378. The answer is c. (*Mengel, pp 273–277.*) The test described in this question is called the straight leg raising test. The test is considered positive when the patient feels pain below the knee when the leg is raised 30°–60°. The positive test indicates nerve root irritation, likely due to a herniated disk. A back strain should not produce a positive straight leg raising test.

A compression fracture may occur suddenly, but would be unlikely in an otherwise healthy young man. Neoplasms and inflammatory conditions would be less likely to occur suddenly.

379. The answer is b. *(Mengel, pp 273–277.)* MRI is indicated for people whose pain persists for more than 6 weeks despite normal radiographs and no response to conservative therapy. Flexion/extension films would not be helpful in identifying more concerning causes of pain. EMG is not indicated without neurological involvement. A bone scan and/or erythrocyte sedimentation rate should be considered in those with symptoms consistent with cancer or infection.

380. The answer is c. *(Mengel, pp 273–277.)* It is recommended that patients with low back pain maintain usual activities, as dictated by pain. Neither prolonged bed rest nor traction has been shown to be effective in returning people to their usual activities sooner. NSAIDs are effective for short-term symptomatic pain relief. Muscle relaxants appear to be effective as well. Opioids may be indicated in pain relief for those who have failed NSAIDs, but are significantly sedating. Steroids can be considered in those who have failed NSAID therapy.

381. The answer is a. *(Mengel, pp 273–277.)* There is strong evidence that individualized exercise programs through physical therapy or an exercise trainer has beneficial effects and can allow most people to perform specific tasks required on a daily basis at home or at work. There is no evidence that antidepressants, steroid injections, traction, and acupuncture provide any additional benefit.

382. The answer is b. *(Mengel, pp 295–300.)* The provocative maneuver described in this question is called Spurling's test. It is positive with nerve root irritation that may accompany a disk herniation. It would not be positive with cervical strain, spondylosis, or arthritis. Torticollis is a sudden onset of unilateral muscular pain, and would also not produce a positive Spurling's test.

383. The answer is b. *(Mengel, pp 295–300.)* The Canadian cervical spine rules help to identify which patients with neck pain require radiographic evaluation. If a patient is unable to rotate his/her neck 45° regardless of pain, x-rays are indicated. MRI, bone scan and DEXA scanning are not indicated in this situation.

384. The answer is b. (*Mengel, pp 429–441.*) Chronic bronchitis is defined as a productive cough lasting 3 consecutive months over 2 consecutive years. Emphysema is generally not a clinical diagnosis, requiring evidence of terminal airway airspace enlargement due to alveoli destruction. Chronic bronchitis and emphysema are the clinical manifestations of COPD. Asthma is a result of airway hyperreactivity, and cannot be assumed given the above history. Bronchiectasis is a destruction of the bronchial walls leads to permanent dilation of the bronchi, with infection as the major cause. Clinical features include a persistent cough with purulent sputum production. Pneumonia would be unlikely given the clinical features described.

385. The answer is e. (*Mengel, pp 429–441.*) Alpha 1-antitrypsin deficiency is a rare genetic abnormality, accounting for less than 1% of the cases of COPD. It should be suspected in people who develop COPD before age 50, especially in nonsmokers, and in people with a family history. The x-ray would show typical emphysematous blebs, especially in the basilar areas. HIV, congestive heart failure and lung cancer are unlikely causes of the x-ray findings described. The patient does not meet the criteria for chronic bronchitis.

386. The answer is e. (*Mengel, pp 429–441.*) The patient described in the question has risk factors and physical stigmata of COPD. Office spirometry is helpful to diagnose COPD and assess its severity. While all the answer choices are common measurements of airflow, the more sensitive measure to diagnose COPD is the FEV_1/FVC ratio. It is considered normal if it is 70% or more of the predicted value based on the patient's gender, age and height. The total lung capacity is not often used in the routine management of COPD, but may be important for restrictive disease.

387. The answer is c. (*Mengel, pp 429–441.*) A number of studies demonstrate that anticholinergic agents produce significantly greater bronchodilation, reduce mucous hypersecretion, have fewer side effects, and less tachycardia than beta-adrenergic agents. Therefore, they are considered the first line therapy for emphysema. The other medications may be used or added, if there is inadequate or suboptimal response.

388. The answer is b. (*Mengel, pp 429–441.*) Theophylline enhances bronchodilation when added to other medications, but also works by enhancing diaphragmatic function and stimulating the respiratory center. It also improves cardiac output, decreases pulmonary vascular resistance, and can improve the perfusion of ischemic cardiac muscle, therefore is of benefit for patients with cor pulmonale or cardiac disease. The therapeutic range is narrow, and is altered by many things making the risk of toxicity high. Toxicity is more likely in the setting of liver disease, and smoking speeds the rate of metabolism.

389. The answer is d. (*Rakel, pp 882–889.*) Weight, diabetes, and hypertension, by themselves, do not indicate the presence or absence of renal insufficiency. However, most cases of chronic renal failure are caused by diabetes and hypertension (60%), so those should be recognized as significant risk factors. The serum creatinine level can be normal in elderly people with chronic renal insufficiency, because they generally have less muscle mass. Therefore, the best indicator of the presence of renal failure is the glomerular filtration rate.

390. The answer is e. (*Rakel, pp 882–889.*) The kidney's role in concentrating and diluting urine is usually retained until the GFR falls below 30% of normal. Therefore, hyponatremia, hyperkalemia, hyperphosphatemia, and metabolic acidosis (due to a fall in plasma bicarbonate) generally occur in later stages of kidney disease. The kidney is the source of erythropoietin, and anemia generally appears when the GFR falls below 60 mL/minute.

391. The answer is c. (*Rakel, pp 882–889.*) The National Kidney Foundation staging system is useful to clinicians as it helps guide appropriate testing and referral for patients with kidney failure. Stage 0 represents people at risk for renal failure, but with a GFR greater than 90 mL/minute. In these people, control of blood pressure and diabetes may forestall the progression to kidney failure. Stage 1 renal failure represents evidence of renal damage (either microalbuminuria or proteinuria), but with a GFR greater than 90 mL/minute. Stage 2 renal failure represents mildly reduced GFR (values between 60–90 mL/minute). In stage 3, the GFR is between 30–59 mL/minute. Stage 4 represents moderate to severe renal failure with GFR levels from 15 to 29 mL/minute, and stage 5 represents severe renal failure with GFR less than 15 mL/minute.

392. The answer is b. (*Rakel, pp 882–889.*) Evidence has shown that ACE inhibitors and angiotensin receptor blockers prevent the evolution of proteinuria and are renal protective. The other medications listed in this question, along with thiazide diuretics, are not renal protective, but may be necessary to achieve optimal blood pressure control (one of the best measures to avoid renal failure).

393. The answer is d. *(Rakel, pp 882–889.)* According to National Kidney Foundation guidelines, this patient has stage 1 renal failure. ACE inhibitors should be added to his regimen to prevent the evolution of microalbuminuria to full blown proteinuria. Improvements in diet and exercise are always appropriate, but should not take the place of the addition of an ACEI. Checking a glycosolated hemoglobin level would not be indicated as a screen for diabetes.

394. The answer is d. *(Rakel, pp 882–889.)* The patient's laboratory values and clinical picture is consistent with moderate renal failure (National Kidney Foundation stage 3). At this point, nephrology referral is indicated. Renal replacement therapy (transplant or dialysis) is indicated for severe renal insufficiency (GFR less than 15 mL/minute).

395. The answer is d. *(Goldberg, Chopra)* There are many physical manifestations of cirrhosis, and some can help determine the underlying cause of liver disease. Spider angiomata and palmar erythema are non-specific, and can be seen with many etiologies. Dupuytren's contractures, testicular atrophy, and parotid gland enlargement are seen more commonly with alcoholic cirrhosis. Splenomegaly is common, especially in patients with cirrhosis from nonalcoholic etiologies.

396. The answer is e. *(Goldberg, Chopra)* Liver tests are followed in patients with cirrhosis to assess severity and progress. While all of the tests above may be abnormal in patients with cirrhosis, bilirubin may be normal if the cirrhosis is well-compensated. Rising serum bilirubin may indicate a poor prognosis in patients with primary biliary cirrhosis.

397. The answer is a. *(Goldberg and Chopra)* Hyponatremia is common in patients with cirrhosis and ascites and is related to the inability to excrete free water. This results from high levels of antidiuretic hormone secretion.

398. The answer is e. *(Goldberg and Chopra)* The gold standard for diagnosing cirrhosis is the examination of the liver following transplantation or autopsy. In clinical practice, cirrhosis is diagnosed with a liver biopsy. The sensitivity of liver biopsy is in between 80–100%. Biopsy is not necessary if the clinical, laboratory, and radiologic data strongly suggest the presence of cirrhosis. This may be the case in a patient with ascites, coagulopathy, and a shrunken nodular appearing liver on ultrasound.

399. The answer is e. (*Goldberg and Chopra*) Determining the cause of liver disease has important implications for treatment. The most important aspect of diagnosing alcoholic liver disease is the documentation of chronic alcohol abuse. However, alcohol use is sometimes denied by the patient. Alcoholic hepatitis is associated with the classic laboratory findings of a disproportionate elevation of AST compared to ALT with both values usually being less than 300 IU/L. This ratio is generally greater than 2.0, a value rarely seen in other forms of liver disease.

400. The answer is e. (*Mengel, pp 442–447.*) Laboratory studies that represent acute hepatocellular injury include AST, ALT, lactate dehydrogenase, and alkaline phosphatase. Laboratory values that represent hepatic function include albumin, bilirubin, and prothrombin time. Tests of hepatic function are more suggestive of chronic disease as opposed to acute injury.

401. The answer is b. (*Mengel, pp 442–447.*) Common hepatotoxic medications include tricyclic antidepressants, muscle relaxants, lipid lowering drugs, antidiabetic agents, antifungal agents, and anticonvulsants. NSAIDs are especially important to avoid because they inhibit platelet function and may exacerbate coagulopathy.

402. The answer is c. (*Mengel, pp 442–447.*) Varicies occur secondary to chronic high pressure in the portal veins. Bleeding from varicies is the most common cause of death in the cirrhotic patients. The other potential causes of death are less common.

403. The answer is b. (*Mengel, pp 442–447.*) Absolute contraindications to liver transplantation include portal vein thrombosis, severe medical illness, malignancy, hepatobiliary sepsis, or lack of patient understanding. Relative contraindications are active alcoholism, HIV or Hepatitis B surface antigen positivity, extensive previous abdominal surgery, and a lack of a personal support system.

404. The answer is d. (*Mengel, pp 447–458.*) Hepatojugular reflux is helpful in differentiating hepatomegaly resulting from heart failure versus other conditions. While compressing the right upper quadrant, the neck veins are observed. This maneuver increases venous return to the heart, and in heart failure patients the jugular veins expand during and immediately after the compression. This is because of the inability of the heart to respond to the increased venous supply.

405. The answer is e. (*Mengel, pp 447–458.*) An S3 gallop occurs from ventricular vibration with rapid diastolic filling. It is therefore best heard in the apical location. Since it is a low-pitched sound, the bell should be used during auscultation. Putting the patient in the 45° left lateral decubitus position doubles the yield.

406. The answer is c. (*Mengel, pp 447–458.*) BNP is elevated in both systolic and diastolic heart failure, and is helpful for distinguishing heart failure from other causes of dyspnea. Wheezes are common with heart failure, as bronchospasm may occur as a consequence of transudate into the alveoli and mucosal congestion. Dullness to percussion occurs with pulmonary edema. A pulmonary embolus may present with an elevated BNP, but a deep venous thrombosis would likely not involve both legs and cause bilateral lower extremity edema. Aspriation would not lead to an increased BNP.

407. The answer is b. (*Mengel, pp 447–458.*) Routine laboratory testing in a person with the new diagnosis of heart failure includes an electrocardiogram, a complete blood count, a urinalysis, serum creatinine, potassium and albumin levels, and thyroid function studies. An echocardiogram is imperative to help identify structural abnormalities of the heart and to measure the ejection fraction. Holter monitoring is not routinely warranted.

408. The answer is b. (*Mengel, pp 447–458.*) The New York Heart Association Functional Classification is important for clinicians to understand, as therapy may change as patients progress from class to class. Class I patients have no limitation of activity. Class II patients have slight limitations, are comfortable at rest, but have fatigue, palpitations, dyspnea, or angina with ordinary activity. Class III patients are also comfortable at rest, but less than ordinary activity causes symptoms. Class IV patients have symptoms at rest, and increased symptoms with even minor activity. There is no "Class V" in this system.

409. The answer is e. (*Mengel, pp 447–458.*) Many noncardiac comorbid conditions may affect the proper diagnosis and clinical course of heart failure. All of the interventions in this question should be done, but only discontinuing alcohol use has actually been shown to improve function significantly. Optimally treating COPD is important, as exacerbations from heart failure are often difficult to distinguish from COPD exacerbations. Optimally treating diabetes and hypertension will mini-mize the negative effects of these conditions on the heart, but will not improve damage already done. Cigarette smoking should be discontin-ued, but generally does not lead to functional improvement. Those with alcoholic cardiomyopathy actually see improvement of the LV function with abstinence.

410. The answer is d. (*Mengel, pp 447–458.*) Some patients have diffi-culty maintaining optimal fluid balance, and a second diuretic is needed. In this case, adding metolazone can significantly increase diuresis in the out-patient treatment of heart failure with volume overload. Prolonged therapy should be avoided. Hydrocholorozide would not enhance diuresis, nor would triamterene. Spironolactone can be used, but is usually only consid-ered for NYHA Class III or IV patients or those with a serum potassium level less than 5.0 mmol/L.

411. The answer is a. (*Mengel, pp 447–458.*) Many clinical trials have shown that ACEIs decrease symptoms, improve quality of life, decrease hos-pitalizations, and reduce mortality in patients with NYHA Class II–IV heart failure. In addition, they slow the progression to heart failure among asymp-tomatic patients with left ventricular systolic dysfunction. All patients with heart failure should be prescribed an ACEI unless they have a contraindica-tion. Beta-blockers are helpful, but not necessarily as a first line agent. Nitrates and hydralazine can be used in patients who do not tolerate ACEIs, as can angiotensin II receptor blockers. Some calcium-channel blockers (nifedipine, diltiazem, and nicardipine) may worsen systolic dysfunction.

412. The answer is b. (*Mengel, pp 447–458.*) ACEIs work to decrease pre-load and afterload in patients with heart failure, and should be considered the first-line therapy. In patients unable to tolerate ACEIs, angiotensin II receptor blockers are a reasonable alternative. In fact, studies are showing mortality reductions equivalent to ACEIs. Another alternative would be the combination of hydralazine and isosorbide dinitrate, but compliance with this regimen is poor. Switching to another ACEI would be inappropriate in light of the fact that the patient experienced angioedema with lisinopril. Nifedipine can worsen symptoms. Beta-blockers are use adjunctively, not alternatively. There is no indication to use clonidine in the patient described.

413. The answer is c. (*Mengel, pp 447–458.*) Beta-blockers inhibit the adverse effects of sympathetic nervous system activation in heart failure patients. Studies have shown that three beta-blockers (bisoprolol, metoprolol, and carvedilol) can reduce symptoms, improve quality of life and reduce mortality. Adding diuretics does not change mortality. Nifedipine can worsen symptoms. Digoxin improves symptoms, but does not decrease mortality.

414. The answer is e. *(Rakel, pp 1071–1077.)* Loss of synapses is believed to be the critical pathologic substrate of Alzheimer's disease. Brain atrophy, destruction of neurons, and shrinkage of neurons occur commonly in the disease, but are also seen in elderly patients without the disease.

415. The answer is b. *(Rakel, pp 1071–1077.)* The decline in cholinergic activity associated with Alzheimer's is well-documented, and is the basis for the approved treatments for the disease. Additional changes have been noted, including deficiencies in glutamate, norepinepherine, serotonin, somatostatin, and corticotrophin-releasing factors, but these are less consistent.

416. The answer is d. Dementia is often difficult to distinguish from delirium or depression in the elderly. However, delirium is generally acute in onset and associated with a loss of concentration. Dementia's onset is insidious, and concentration is less likely to be a problem. Depression is associated with psychomotor slowing, while dementia is generally not. While people with dementia may complain of memory loss, it is far more likely that the patient's family will complain of the patient having memory loss in dementia. Depressed patients usually present themselves complaining of memory loss. Depressed and delirious patients will generally show poor effort in testing, while demented patients will generally display good effort, but get wrong answers.

417. The answer is e. *(Rakel, pp 1071–1077.)* Often, memory disturbances are the presenting symptom in Alzheimer's disease. Remote memories are well-preserved initially, with the ability to recall new information being lost early in the illness. Decreased conversational output is also noted early. Decreased ability to recognize and draw complex figures is an early sign of problems, as is the loss of the ability to calculate. Social propriety and interpersonal skills often remain strikingly preserved until late in the illness.

418. The answer is d. *(Rakel, pp 1071–1077.)* In the past, it was thought that vascular dementia (multi-infarct dementia, or that occurring after a stroke) was common. This is because MRI scans from demented patients often show changes consistent with small-vessel ischemic disease. Those changes are not seen as being significant without the appropriate clinical picture. The typical history would include episodic abrupt changes, as described in this question, and imaging findings consistent with ischemia. Alzheimer's disease, Parkinson's disease, and alcoholic dementia would likely be more insidious in onset. Depression is often a problem in the elderly, and may be mistaken for dementia. It would not follow the described course, however.

419. The answer is d. (*Rakel, pp 1071–1077.*) The routine evaluation in patients with dementia includes a complete blood count, a chemistry panel, thyroid function testing, a vitamin B-12 level, and an MRI of the brain. When indicated based on clinical findings, the evaluation can include an erythrocyte sedimentation rate, urinalysis, toxicology screen, chest x-ray, heavy metal screen, HIV screen, syphilis serology, CSF evaluation, and an EEG.

420. The answer is e. (*Rakel, pp 1071–1077.*) Three cholinesterase inhibitors are approved for the treatment of Alzheimer's disease. They include donepezil (Aricept), galantamine (Reminyl), and rivastigmine (Exelon). They reduce the metabolism of acetylcholinesterase, thereby prolonging its action at cholinergic synapses. They are associated with modest improvements in cognition, behavior, activities of daily living and global measurements of functioning. However, they do not slow the progression of neurodegeneration.

421. The answer is d. (*Rakel, pp 1071–1077. Mengel, pp 459–476.*) The patient described has dementia of Lewy body (DLB) type. This begins similarly to Alzheimer's disease, but then patients develop complex visual hallucinations and spontaneous signs of Parkinsonism. Patients with Alzheimer's dementia develop delusions, but rarely have hallucinations. Antipsychotics should be avoided in this type of dementia, unless absolutely necessary, as there is concern for long-term neurological damage. DLB responds to cholinesterase inhibitors, and the other medications listed are safe if used appropriately.

422. The answer is b. (*South-Paul, pp 424–442.*) The American Diabetes Association recommends screening all persons older than 45 years old for diabetes every 3 years. Screens should start earlier in people with risk factors including a family history of diabetes in a first degree relative, hypertension, obesity, high risk ethnic groups (African American, Hispanic, Native American), a previous history of impaired glucose tolerance, abnormal lipids (especially elevated triglycerides and low HDL), and women with a history of gestational diabetes or a birth of a child greater than 9 lb. Multiple screens are available. Random glucose is easy, but has low specificity. A 2-hour glucose tolerance test is more specific, but is more costly and time consuming. A 1-hour glucose tolerance test is generally used for screening pregnant women, with a 3-hour glucose tolerance test being used for those that are positive. Urinalyses are highly specific, but has low sensitivity. Fasting glucose is more accurate, and is generally recommended.

423. The answer is c. (*South-Paul, pp 424–442.*) The diagnosis of diabetes may be made by two separate random glucose measurements more than 200 mg/dL with classic signs of diabetes (polydipsia, polyuria, polyphagia, weight loss), a fasting glucose greater than 126 mg/dL, or a glucose reading greater than 200 mg/dL 2 hours after a 75-g glucose load.

424. The answer is a. (*South-Paul, pp 424–442.*) In the past, young adults diagnosed with diabetes were primarily type 1. However, the epidemic of obesity in the United States has increased the rate of type 2 diabetes in people less than 20 years old from 5% to 30% over the last decade. C-peptide is cleaved from natively produced insulin. In people with type 1 diabetes, c-peptide levels should be low. Microalbuminuria, markedly elevated Hemoglobin A1C and peripheral neuropathy can all occur in type 1 or type 2 diabetes.

425. The answer is b. (*South-Paul, pp 424–442.*) Of the 300,000 patients in the United States with end-stage renal disease (ESRD), one-third of those have their disease due to diabetic nephropathy. While the other listed answers may cause ESRD, diabetes is the most common cause.

426. The answer is d. (*South-Paul, pp 424–442.*) The first indication of renal compromise in diabetics is an increase in glomerular filtration rate. Renal lesions develop, and are followed by microalbuminuria. Uncorrected, this can lead to macroalbuminuria, then renal failure. ACE inhibitors have been shown to decrease end-stage renal disease and death by 41% in diabetics. Lifestyle changes including glucose control, weight loss, and decreased protein intake can help, but experts agree that the benefits of ACE inhibitors are well-documented. Nephrology referral would be indicated if the creatinine becomes elevated, or in the face of macroalbuminuria or microalbuminuria despite maximal therapy. Even in patients who are normotensive, low dose ACE inhibitors are beneficial in the face of microalbuminuria.

427. The answer is a. (*South-Paul, pp 424–442.*) Diabetic retinopathy is the leading cause of blindness in the United States. The risk increases with the length of time that the patient has had diabetes, and the condition worsens with increasing hemoglobin A1C levels. In type 2 diabetics, it can be seen at diagnosis. Aspirin has no effect on eye complications. It follows a predictable pattern, with mild background abnormalities followed by increased vascular permeability and hemorrhage. Proliferative changes occur late in the course.

428. The answer is a. (*South-Paul, pp 424–442.*) Heart disease is the leading cause of death in diabetic patients. The prevalence of fatal and nonfatal coronary disease is 2–20 times higher in diabetic patients than in nondiabetics. There has been an overall decline in the incidence of heart disease in people in the United States, but not in diabetics. While pneumonia and infections are more common in diabetics, they do not surpass heart disease as a cause of death.

429. The answer is c. (*South-Paul, pp 424–442.*) ACE Inhibitors are clearly the first choice for blood pressure control in diabetic patients. They control blood pressure effectively, help prevent progression of renal disease, and are indicated in the presence of coronary disease and congestive heart failure. The other listed medications can be added for improved control if needed.

430. The answer is b. (*South-Paul, pp 424–442.*) Statins are the drug of choice in treating hyperlipidemia in diabetes. They have been shown to decrease the risk of coronary events and are excellent in lowering LDL. They do have less effect on the triglyceride levels, but in many patients, the decrease is enough to get patients to goal. Niacin will decrease triglycerides, raise HDL and lower LDL, but may increase insulin resistance. Niacin is often used in combination with a statin or alone in patients with statin side effects. Fibric acid derivatives lower triglycerides and raise HDL, but have minimal effects on LDL. Bile acid resins sequester bile acids in the GI tract. They can increase triglyceride levels, and are generally not used in diabetics.

431. The answer is a. (*South-Paul, pp 424–442.*) Glycemic control is dependent on the total caloric intake, not the type of calorie taken in. Low carbohydrate and high protein diets have not been shown to improve glucose control more than weight loss from other methods. Sucrose does not need to be eliminated, but it may raise blood sugar more quickly after ingestion. Formal dietary programs are not more likely to produce long-term sustainable results unless exercise is a large component of the plan. Increased fiber does improve glycemic control.

432. The answer is d. *(South-Paul, pp 424–442.)* Oral therapy for type 2 diabetes can be complicated. No evidence supports changing sulfonylureas when one isn't adequately controlling glucose levels. Biguanides act to decrease glucose output from the liver, and can decrease hemoglobin A1C by 1.5–2%. However, biguanides should not be used if creatinine is higher than 1.5 mg/dL. Meglitinides increase insulin secretion, and should only be taken before meals. They can reduce the hemoglobin A1C by 0.5–2% and are most valuable if fasting sugar is adequate, but postprandial sugars are high. Since they increase insulin levels, they are more effective when used in combination with a medication that has a different mechanism of action. They are excreted in the liver, therefore are safe in renal failure. Thiazolidinediones decrease insulin resistance and are an excellent choice for those with insulin insensitivity. Alpha-glucosidase inhibitors inhibit the absorption of carbohydrates in the gut and can decrease the hemoglobin A1C by 0.7–1%. They should be avoided if creatinine more than 2.0 mg/dL.

433. The answer is d. *(Hinnen)* The recently approved incretin-mimetic agent exenatide is indicated for patients who have not achieved adequate glycemic control with oral agents that include metformin and sulfonylureas. Studies with thiazolidinediones are forthcoming. Patients taking exenatide experience modest reductions in weight and in HbA_{1C}. Incretin-mimetic agents have multiple mechanisms of action for the treatment of type 2 diabetes mellitus, including enhancement of glucose-dependent insulin secretion, suppression of inappropriately elevated glucagon, slowing of gastric emptying, and decreased food intake.

434. The answer is b. *(MacFarlane)* Thiazolidinediones have been associated with an increased risk of peripheral edema. A meta-analysis was performed to assess the overall risk for developing edema secondary to TZD. Odds ratios were generated by pooling estimates across the studies. The pooled odds ratio for TZD induced edema was 2.26 (95% CI: 2.02–2.53). The results yielded a higher risk for developing edema with rosiglitazone (3.75 [2.70–5.20]) compared to pioglitazone (2.42 [1.90–3.08]). This meta-analysis demonstrates at least a twofold increase in the risk for developing edema with a TZD agent. The risk appears to be greater with rosiglitazone than with pioglitazone.

Despite an increase in fluid-related events, recent studies suggest that individuals with type 2 diabetes mellitus and heart failure (New York Heart Association grade I/II) can be treated with thiazolidinediones with appropriate monitoring and adjustment of heart failure therapies.

435. The answer is e. (*Drucker*) Glucagon-like peptide 1 (GLP-1) is a gut-derived incretin hormone that stimulates insulin and suppresses glucagon secretion, inhibits gastric emptying, and reduces appetite and food intake. Therapeutic approaches for enhancing incretin action include degradation-resistant GLP-1 receptor agonists (incretin mimetics), and inhibitors of dipeptidyl peptidase-4 (DPP-4) activity (incretin enhancers). Orally administered DPP-4 inhibitors, such as sitagliptin reduce HbA1c by 0.5–1.0%, with few adverse events and no weight gain. These new classes of antidiabetic agents, and incretin mimetics and enhancers, also expand beta-cell mass in preclinical studies.

436. The answer is a. (*Mengel, pp 476–484.*) It is important to thoroughly understand the action of the different types of insulin preparations in order to make therapeutic decisions about diabetic patients and their control. Aspart has the most rapid onset of action, between 15–30 minutes. Regular insulin has an onset between 30–60 minutes. Lente's onset is between 1–2 hours, as is Lantus'. Ultralente's onset is between 2–4 hours.

437. The answer is c. (*Mengel, pp 476–484.*) It is important to thoroughly understand the action of the different types of insulin preparations in order to make therapeutic decisions about diabetic patients and their control. Aspart's activity peaks early, between 30–60 minutes after injection. Regular insulin peaks between 2–3 hours after injection. Lente's peak is between 4–8 hours, and Ultralente's peak is between 8–20 hours. One of the important things to remember about Lantus is that it does not have a peak.

438. The answer is d. (*Mengel, pp 476–484.*) It is important to thoroughly understand the action of the different types of insulin preparations in order to make therapeutic decisions about diabetic patients and their control. Aspart's duration of action is between 3–5 hours. Regular insulin lasts between 4–12 hours. Lente's duration is between 10–20 hours, and Lantus' duration is around 24 hours. The longest duration is with Ultralente, which lasts 24–32 hours.

439. The answer is c. *(Mengel, pp 476–484.)* There are many methods for determining the appropriate amount of insulin that will be required in type 1 diabetics. One way is to determine the total amount of insulin used while hospitalized, and divide that dose during the day. Two-thirds of the total insulin should be given in the morning, with the remaining one-third in the evening. Each time the patient receives insulin, 75% of the dose should be NPH, and 25% should be regular. In this question, the patient needed 100 units of insulin. Of this, 67 units should be given in the morning, and 33 units should be given in the evening. Of the morning dose, 75% should be NPH. Seventy-five percent of 67 units equals to 50. Therefore, the patient should get 50 units of NPH in the morning and 17 units of regular.

440. The answer is c. *(Mengel, pp 476–484.)* When using Lantus and Lispro, approximately 40–50% of the total daily insulin requirements should be given as Lantus, with the remaining 50–60% of insulin given as Lispro before each meal, based on a preprandial glucose reading.

441. The answer is b. *(Mengel, pp 476–484.)* Patients with type 2 diabetes may require insulin therapy if diet, exercise and oral hypoglycemic agent do not provide appropriate control. A low dose of NPH is commonly used, estimating 0.1 unit/kg of body weight, as an addition to the current regimen.

442. The answer is b. *(Koski)* Metformin should be withheld before a procedure with radiocontrast dye, as contrast-induced nephropathy may predispose to developing lactic acidosis if a patient is taking concurrent metformin. It should also be withheld for surgery. It can be restarted immediately after surgery if the person's renal function is normal and his or her condition is stable.

443. The answer is b. *(Mengel, pp 484–499.)* Alcohol, in moderation, raises HDL cholesterol. Alternatively, cigarette smoking decreases HDL. Being overweight or obese decreases HDL, but weight loss may not raise HDL. Low dietary intake of cholesterol has no impact on HDL. Stress can markedly increase LDL cholesterol, but will not impact HDL.

444. The answer is a. *(Mengel, pp 484–499.)* Blood lipids change acutely in response to food intake. The triglyceride level is lowest in the fasting state, and rises by an average of 50 mg/dL portprandially. As the TG level rises, the total and LDL cholesterol each fall. Thus total and LDL cholesterol tend to be higher when fasting. HDL varies little whether fasting or not.

445. The answer is c. (*Mengel, pp 484–499.*) Of all the lipid values, HDL is the single best predictor of an adverse outcome. However, high HDL does not guarantee immunity from coronary artery disease. C-reactive protein levels predict risk for myocardial infarction and stroke even better than LDL levels do, but are not as beneficial as HDL.

446. The answer is d. (*Mengel, pp 484–499.*) Smoking cessation increases HDL by 5–10 mg/dL, but does not affect LDL, VLDL, or triglycerides.

447. The answer is b. (*Mengel, pp 484–499.*) Aspirin blocks much of the flushing that is associated with sustained release niacin preparations. Taking niacin at night, with food, on an empty stomach or with milk will not impact the side effects.

448. The answer is e. (*Mengel, pp 484–499.*) Pravastatin (Pravachol), fluvastatin (Lescol), and rosuvastatin (Crestor) are not metabolized by the cytochrome P-450 3A4 enzyme system and therefore have less potential for drug interactions. Atorvastatin (Lipitor), simvastatin (Zocor), lovastatin (Mevacor) either alone or in combination are more likely to cause interactions.

449. The answer is e. (*Mengel, pp 484–499.*) Fish oil is high in omega-3 fatty acids and have been shown to be beneficial in lowering cholesterol. Fish oils work by decreasing secretion of triglycerides by the liver.

450. The answer is b. (*Mengel, pp 484–499.*) Gemfibrozil changes the hepatic metabolism of lipoproteins and is a logical choice for the patient with low HDL and elevated triglycerides.

451. The answer is d. (*Mengel, pp 484–499.*) Ezetemibe (Zetia) lowers cholesterol by interfering with the absorption of cholesterol in the gut. Used alone, it lowers LDL and triglycerides only modestly. When added to a low-dose statin, the combination lowers LDL as much as the maximum statin dose, but its combined use with a low dose statin may produce fewer adverse effects.

452. The answer is d. (*Taylor, pp 360–367.*) HIV results should always be given during a face-to-face interview. Even in a low risk patient, if the results are positive, it represents a life-changing event. It is important to reassure the patient regarding possibly inappropriate assumptions about HIV infection. Sending the results via mail, or discussing the results on the telephone would not be appropriate. Even with negative results, it is important to discuss risk reduction with the patient and develop a plan to prevent future exposure.

453. The answer is d. *(Taylor, pp 360–367.)* Testing to establish the diagnosis of HIV infection usually requires an ELISA followed by a confirmatory Western blot of immunofluroescent antibody test. However, there is a "window period" of several weeks to 3 months between the infection and seroconversion when these tests may be negative. During this time, patients may be viremic and infectious, but not have sufficient levels of antibodies to result in positive tests. If there is strong clinical suspicion, plasma HIV RNA should be ordered. P24 antigen assay can be checked, but has a higher false-positive rate.

454. The answer is c. *(Taylor, pp 360–367.)* Vaccinations appropriate for HIV infected individuals include Hepatitis A and B, if there is no evidence of prior exposure and immunity. In the case described the patient has prior exposure and immunity, since his antibody tests are positive. Yearly influenza and a one-time pneumococcal vaccination should be administered. Live vaccines should not be administered, so MMR and oral polio should not be given. Polio vaccination for HIV infected persons should be with the inactivated (intramuscular) preparation.

455. The answer is c. *(Taylor, pp 360–367.)* Usually, induration of 15 mm (10 mm in high risk patients) indicates a positive test. In HIV infected individuals, 5 mm is considered a positive test. PPD tests should be placed annually in HIV infected patients, as there is an increased risk of progression from latent to active TB in infected individuals.

456. The answer is a. *(Taylor, pp 360–367.)* Prophylaxis against *Mycobacterium avium* complex (MAC) should be instituted once the patient's CD4 count drops below 50. Prophylaxis against *Pneumocystis carinii* pneumonia should be considered once the CD4 count drops below 200. Primary prophylaxis is not indicated for fungal infections, herpes simplex, herpes zoster, or cytomegalovirus.

457. The answer is c. *(Taylor, pp 360–367.)* The x-ray shown is suspicious for *Pneumocystis carinii* pneumonia, and treatment should be started immediately. The treatment of choice is trimethoprim-sulfamethoxazole

(TMP-SMX) for 3 weeks. However, if the PaO$_2$ falls below 70 mm Hg, the patient should receive concurrent steroids.

458. The answer is e. *(Mengel, pp 499–507.)* The patient described above has stage 2 hypertension (systolic blood pressure greater or equal to 160 mm Hg, or diastolic blood pressure greater or equal to 90 mm Hg). Since lifestyle modifications have not helped, the next step is to institute drug therapy. JNC 7 guidelines state that in patients with stage 2 hypertension, two-drug combination therapy is indicated. The most common regimen would be a thiazide diuretic along with either an ACE inhibitor, ARB, beta-blocker, or calcium-channel blocker.

459. The answer is d. *(Mengel, pp 499–507.)* When examining a hypertensive patient, the physician should be alert for signs of end-organ damage and possible causes of secondary hypertension. Signs of end-organ damage include arteriolar narrowing, hemorrhages, exudates or papilledema, carotid bruits or jugular venous distension, a loud second heart sound or precordial heave, arrhythmias, absent peripheral pulses, and peripheral edema, just to name a few. Signs suggestive of secondary hypertension include abdominal or flank masses (polycystic kidneys), absence of femoral pulses (coarctation of the aorta), tachycardia/flushing/diaphoresis (pheochromocytoma), abdominal bruits (renal artery stenosis), pigmented striae (Cushing's syndrome), or an enlarged thyroid gland (hyperthyroidism).

460. The answer is c. *(Mengel, pp 499–507.)* Baseline laboratory screening is important to assess for end-organ damage and identify patients at high risk for cardiovascular complications. The routine tests for a newly diagnosed hypertensive patient include: hemoglobin and hematocrit, potassium, creatinine, fasting glucose, calcium, a fasting lipid profile, urinalysis, and a resting electrocardiogram. Other tests are not indicated unless physical examination or history makes them likely to be positive.

461. The answer is c. *(Mengel, pp 499–507.)* The patient described in the question has symptoms consistent with pheochromocytoma. The best test to rule this out is urinary metanephrines and vanillymandelic acid levels. A chest x-ray would be helpful if coarctation of the aorta were suspected. A captopril renal scan or renal magnetic resonance angiography would evaluate renal artery stenosis. Plasma renin activity levels would identify primary aldosteronism, and an echocardiogram would help to identify left ventricular hypertrophy or systolic dysfunction.

462. The answer is b. (*Mengel, pp 499–507.*) The patient described in the question has physical examination findings consistent with renal artery stenosis. A captopril renal scan or renal magnetic resonance angiography would evaluate this. Urinary metanephrines and vanillylmandelic acid levels would help rule out pheochromocytoma. A chest x-ray would be helpful if coarctation of the aorta were suspected. An aortic CT would help to or quantify an aortic aneurysm, and an echocardiogram would help to identify left ventricular hypertrophy or systolic dysfunction.

463. The answer is b. (*Mengel, pp 499–507.*) While all of the interventions listed in this question have the potential to lower systolic blood pressure, the DASH diet (described in the landmark study, Dietary Approaches to Stop Hypertension) has been shown to lower blood pressure the most. The diet is high in potassium, calcium, and magnesium. The study found that diets high in fruits and vegetables, with a reduced content of saturated and total fat can lower systolic blood pressure by 8–14 mm Hg. A 10% weight loss will lower blood pressure by 5–10 mm Hg. Sodium restriction will lower blood pressure 2–8 mm Hg. Regular aerobic activity is also beneficial, lowering blood pressure by 4–9 mm Hg, and limiting alcohol can lower systolic blood pressure by 2–4 mm Hg.

464. The answer is a. (*Mengel, pp 499–507.*) The ALLHAT study and a meta-analysis of more than 42 clinical trials has demonstrated that low-dose diuretics are the most effective first-line treatment for preventing the occurrence of cardiovascular morbidity and mortality. If there are no compelling reasons to start another medication, it should be the medication of first choice.

465. The answer is b. (*Mengel, pp 499–507.*) The PROGRESS study (Perindopril Protection against Recurrent Stroke Study) found that an ACE inhibitor and diuretic in combination are effective in preventing recurrent stroke.

466. The answer is b. (*Mengel, pp 499–507.*) Several clinical trials have documented the benefit of ACE inhibitors in patients with hypertension and chronic kidney disease. Angiotension receptor blockers are also beneficial.

467. The answer is e. (*Mengel, pp 499–507.*) According to JNC 7 guidelines, if the initial agent does not control blood pressure sufficiently, a second agent of a different class should be added. Keeping both agents at lower doses will decrease side effects. ACE inhibitors and diuretics work well together with a relatively low incidence of side effects.

468. The answer is b. (*Mengel, pp 508–515.*) Atypical angina occurs when the patient experiences pain that has the quality and characteristics of angina, or occurs with exertion, but not both. For example, atypical angina may be a sense of heaviness not consistently related to exertion or relieved by rest, or it may be pain with an atypical character (sharp or stabbing) but predictably brought on by exercise and relieved by rest. Classic angina has both features. Anginal equivalent occurs when dyspnea is the sole or major manifestation. Nonanginal pain has neither the quality nor the precipitants of angina. "Atypical nonanginal pain" is not a term used to describe chest pain.

469. The answer is c. (*Mengel, pp 508–515.*) An aginal equivalent occurs when a patient has no chest pain, but has other symptoms of cardiac ischemia (e.g., dyspnea) that is predictably precipitated by exertion and relieved by rest. Atypical angina occurs when the patient experiences pain that has the quality and characteristics of angina, or occurs with exertion, but not both. Nonanginal pain has neither the quality nor the precipitants of angina. "Atypical nonanginal pain" is not a term used to describe chest pain.

470. The answer is d. (*Mengel, pp 508–515.*) Nonanginal pain has neither the quality nor the precipitating features of angina. Typical descriptive terms of nonanginal pain include "stabbing," "shooting," "knifelike," "jabbing," and "tingling." Atypical angina occurs when the patient experiences pain that has the quality and characteristics of angina, or occurs with exertion, but not both. Anginal equivalent occurs when dyspnea is the sole or major manifestation. "Atypical nonanginal pain" is not a term used to describe chest pain.

471. The answer is b. (*Mengel, pp 508–515.*) The standard provocative test for ischemic heart disease is an exercise treadmill test. However, certain ECG abnormalities make the standard ETT unreadable. These include left ventricular hypertrophy with strain, left bundle branch block (shown in the question), and ST segment baseline abnormalities in the precordial leads. In this case, a thallium ETT is preferred, as long as the patient can exercise.

472. The answer is d. (*Mengel, pp 508–515.*) Poor prognostic signs in an exercise treadmill test include failure to complete stage II of a Bruce protocol, failure to achieve a heart rate greater than 120 beats per minute (off beta-blockers), onset of ST segment depression at a heart rate less than 120 beats per minute, having ST segment depression greater than 2.0 mm, having ST segment depression lasting more than 6 minutes into recovery, poor systolic blood pressure response to exercise, angina or ventricular tachycardia with exercise, and ST segment depression in multiple leads.

473. The answer is e. (*Mengel, pp 508–515.*) Tolerance is the most significant issue to consider when using nitrates for stable angina. Tolerance develops rapidly when long-acting nitrates are given. When using a patch, it is important to have intervals of 10–12 hours without the patch to retain the antianginal effect. Headache and fatigue may be important side effects, but are more of a nuisance than an important consideration. The medications can be used with beta-blockers and calcium-channel blockers.

474. The answer is c. (*Mengel, pp 508–515.*) All beta-blockers, regardless of their selectivity, are equally effective in treating angina. About 20% of patients do not respond. The dose should be adjusted to achieve a heart rate of 50–60 beats per minute.

475. The answer is d. (*Taylor, pp 455–458.*) Family physicians should be familiar with the use of body mass indices as an indicator of obesity and subsequent health risks. The BMI is determined by dividing the patient's weight in kilograms by the square of the height in meters. A BMI greater than 26 is classified as overweight. A BMI greater than 30 is considered obese, and a BMI greater than 40 is considered morbidly obese.

476. The answer is a. (*Taylor, pp 455–458.*) Secondary causes of obesity are rare, but should be considered in the differential diagnosis for obesity. All of the answers to the question are possible secondary causes; but given the patient's irregular menstrual periods, acne, and hirsuitism, polycystic ovary syndrome is more likely.

477. The answer is b. (*Taylor, pp 455–458.*) There are several well-known health complications of obesity. They include hypertension, diabetes, cancers (most notably breast cancer), dyslipidemias, arthritis, depression, cholelithiasis, coronary artery disease, and sleep apnea among others. Hypothyroidism and Cushing's disease may be secondary causes of obesity, but are not consequences of obesity. Asthma has not been linked to obesity, but the lack of exercise in some patients with asthma may predispose persons to becoming overweight. Osteoporosis risk is not increased in obese people.

478. The answer is b. *(Taylor, pp 455–458.)* When discussing diet plans, it is important to ensure patients have realistic expectations regarding outcomes to avoid frustration and burnout. There are 3500 calories in a pound. All things being equal, diminishing food intake by 500 calories per day will result in weight loss of 1 lb per week.

479. The answer is e. *(Taylor, pp 455–458.)* Overweight patients often inquire about the use of medications to enhance weight loss. Some agents may be a helpful adjunct to diet and exercise, but should not be considered the primary solution. Some medications have been approved by the FDA and are not deemed unsafe when used as directed. Short courses of medication may help initiate weight reduction, but do not help in maintaining weight loss. In fact, in all cases, cessation of the drug has been shown to result in rapid accumulation of weight, if lifestyle changes are not maintained. Long courses of medications have not shown to be helpful in maintaining weight loss, and in most studies, weight is regained despite continued use of medication.

480. The answer is d. *(South-Paul, pp 336–347.)* Osteoporosis is due to poor acquisition of bone mass or accelerated bone loss. African Americans are less at risk than Caucasians or Asians. There is no evidence that oral contraceptive use increases risk. Obesity is considered to be protective due to increased estrogen production, as long as the person is not sedentary. Hyperthyroidism is a common cause of accelerated bone loss. Breast-feeding is a significant drain on calcium stores, but studies have shown that the associated bone mineral loss is completely reversed within 12 months of weaning.

481. The answer is a. *(South-Paul, pp 336–347.)* Weight bearing activity is known to retard bone loss. While there have been no randomized clinical trials comparing the effect of various activities on bone mass, recommended activities include walking, jogging, weight lifting, aerobics, stair climbing, field sports, racquet sports, court sports, and dancing. Swimming is questionable, as it is not weight bearing. There is no data on cycling, skating, or skiing.

482. The answer is e. *(South-Paul, pp 336–347.)* Primary osteoporosis refers to deterioration of bone mass not associated with other chronic illnesses or problems. History and physical are neither sensitive enough nor sufficient for the diagnosis of primary osteoporosis. While decreased serum calcium may indicate malabsorption or a vitamin D deficiency, it is not useful as a diagnostic tool for osteoporosis. Measures of bone turnover, like serum human osteocalin levels, are of research interest, but are not useful for screening. Imaging studies are best.

483. The answer is d. (*South-Paul, pp 336–347.*) Plain radiographs are not sensitive enough to diagnose osteoporosis until total density has decreased by 50%. Single and dual photon absorptiometry provide poor resolution and are less accurate than other methods. Dual energy x-ray absorptiometry (DEXA) scanning is most precise and is the test of choice. Quantitative CT scanning is the most sensitive, but exposes patients to significant levels of radiation exposure.

484. The answer is c. (*South-Paul, pp 336–347.*) Bone densitometry provides a T-score (the number of standard deviations above or below the mean matched to YOUNG controls) and a Z-score (the number of standard deviations above or below the mean-matched to age-matched controls). Z-scores are of little value to clinicians. A T-score more than 2.5 standard deviations below the mean (a score of –2.5 or lower) indicates osteoporosis.

485. The answer is b. (*South-Paul, pp 336–347.*) Absolute contraindications to estrogen replacement therapy include a history of breast cancer or other estrogen-dependent cancer, undiagnosed or abnormal genital bleeding, and a history or an active thromboembolic disorder. Relative contraindications include migraine, a history of thromboembolism, familial hypertriglyceridemia, uterine leiomyoma, uterine cancer, gallbladder disease, a strong family history of breast cancer, chronic hepatic dysfunction, and endometriosis.

486. The answer is c. (*South-Paul, pp 336–347.*) Calcitonin directly inhibits osteoclastic bone resorption and is considered a reasonable treatment alternative for patients with established osteoporosis in whom estrogen replacement therapy is not recommended. It has the unique characteristic of producing an analgesic effect with respect to bone pain and is often prescribed for patients who have suffered an acute osteoporotic fracture.

487. The answer is c. (*South-Paul, pp 336–347.*) Bisphosphonates work by binding to the bone surface and inhibiting osteoclastic activity. Vitamin D increases absorption of calcium in the GI tract. Estrogen and selective estrogen receptor modulators (raloxifene or Evista) work by blocking the activity of cytokines. Fluoride stimulates osteoblasts, but does not result in the formation of normal bone.

488. The answer is b. (*South-Paul, pp 599–609.*) Depression is commonly seen in primary care settings. In fact, it is estimated that only about 20% of depression-related health care occurs in mental health care settings. Nonpsychiatrists write approximately 80% of the prescriptions for antidepressants. Patients with major depressive disorder often present with vague physical symptoms rather than emotional complaints. To make the diagnosis of depression using DSM criteria, the patient must describe either depressed mood for most of the day nearly every day for at least 2 weeks, or loss of interest in usually enjoyable activities. Irritable mood may take the place of depressed mood to make the diagnosis as well. In addition to one of those two symptoms, the patient must experience other symptoms of depression, including sleep changes, feelings of guilt or worthlessness, loss of energy, loss of concentration, change in appetite, psychomotor speeding or slowing, or suicidal thoughts, plans or intent.

489. The answer is a. (*South-Paul, pp 599–609. Mengel, pp 637–645.*) All of the answers to this question would be considered optimal first-line agents for depression, in terms of patient acceptance of side effects, safety, and quantity/quality of clinical trials data available for review. However, those medications that impact the serotonin system have a rather high incidence of sexual side effects (up to 20% in some estimates). Citalopram, fluoxetine, and sertraline are all selective serotonin reuptake inhibitors, and venlafaxine is both a serotonin and norepinephrine reuptake inhibitor. Bupropion is a dopamine and norepinephrine reuptake inhibitor, and therefore is less likely to cause sexual side effects.

490. The answer is d. (*Mengel, pp 637–645.*) Physicians have various treatment options for depression. Studies have shown that the combination of medication and therapy offer the best treatment outcomes. However, antidepressants alone are effective in about 50–60% of patients with major depression. If a patient fails to respond to one medication, he/she may respond to another. At least 80% of patients with major depression will respond to at least one antidepressant medication. In order to prevent relapse, treatment should continue for 6–9 months. Electroconvulsive therapy (ECT) has a high rate of therapeutic success, but is reserved for those who do not respond to other modalities of treatment.

491. The answer is e. (*Mengel, pp 637–645.*) While many of the newer antidepressants are well-tolerated, physicians should be familiar with the adverse effects and contraindications for their use. Nefazodone should not be used in patients with liver disease. Hypertension is a relative contraindication to venlafaxine. Patients experiencing hypersomnia and motor retardation should avoid nefazodone and mirtazapine. Patients who report agitation and insomnia should avoid bupropion and venlafaxine. Mirtazapine and tricyclic antidepressants are less preferred for patients with obesity. Bupropion is contraindicated for patients with seizure disorder.

492. The answer is a. (*South-Paul, pp 610–621. Mengel, pp 604–612.*) Anxiety disorders encompass several clinical conditions including generalized anxiety disorder, panic disorder, the phobias, obsessive-compulsive disorder, and posttraumatic stress disorder. Conversion disorder is not classified as an anxiety disorder, and involves an unintentionally produced motor or sensory function deficit, preceded by conflict or stress. Somatization disorder involves a history of many medical complaints for which treatment is sought that cannot be explained fully by a known medical condition, and is also not classified as an anxiety disorder. Anorexia is classified as an eating disorder, and histrionic personality disorder is a classified among the personality disorders, and involves a dramatic, attention-seeking, and emotional patient.

493. The answer is d. (*Mengel, pp 645–654.*) Eating disorders are psychological disorders in which the person afflicted has an altered perception of body weight or shape and disturbances of eating behavior. Distinguishing between anorexia and bulimia may be important from a treatment standpoint. Some characteristics are common to both eating disorders, while other characteristics may help to differentiate them. Both disorders involve self-evaluation that is unduly influenced by body weight and/or shape. While binge eating or purging are considered characteristics of bulimia, there is a binge eating/purging subtype of anorexia that involves that behavior as well. Both bulimics and binge eating/purging subtypes of anorexics may use diuretics, enemas, and laxatives. Both engage in inappropriate behaviors to prevent weight gain. However, bulimics sense a lack of control over eating during episodes of binging, while anorexics often feel a strong sense of control. This is a characteristic that may help distinguish the two.

494. The answer is c. (*Mengel, pp 612–629.*) The etiology of ADHD is not entirely clear, but genetic factors seem to play a role. Environmental factors including environmental exposure to allergens and toxins have been studied, but do not play a role. The major risk factor for the development of ADHD is family history. Rates of ADHD can be as high as 30% in siblings of an affected individual, and 50% in at least one parent. Low self-esteem and academic underachievement are considered comorbid conditions, but are not considered risk factors.

495. The answer is b. (*Mengel, pp 612–629.*) Of children diagnosed with ADHD, up to 60% will continue to exhibit symptoms into adulthood. In adults, symptoms of ADHD may be more subtle, and symptoms may actually change. Hyperactivity may be replaced with restlessness, and impulsivity may be replaced with inability to control emotions or social inappropriateness. Sleep and appetite disturbances in adults should alert the physician to the possibility of another disorder, especially depression.

496. The answer is c. (*Mengel, pp 612–629.*) Stimulants reduce symptoms of hyperactivity, impulsivity, and inattention. The mechanism of action is thought to be by inhibition of dopamine and norepinephrine reuptake. Approximately 70% of children respond to a specific stimulant, and 90% will respond to at least one stimulant. A positive response to stimulant medication is not diagnostic for ADHD. As children and adults without ADHD who take stimulants demonstrate improvement in attention, concentration, and memory tasks.

497. The answer is a. (*South-Paul, pp 443–461.*) The most common cause of thyroiditis is chronic lymphocytic thyroiditis (also called Hashimoto's thyroiditis). It is the most common cause of goiter in the United States. Generally seen in middle-aged women, this generally presents with enlargement of the thyroid, and most often there is associated tenderness. Subacute lymphocytic thyroiditis is less common, and although an acute increase in thyroid size is seen, it is generally nontender. Subacute granulomatous thyroiditis usually follows a viral illness and is also associated with a mildly painful gland. Suppurative thyroiditis is rare, and is associated with fever, a swollen thyroid and clinical manifestations of a bacterial illness. Invasive fibrous thyroiditis presents as a gradually increasing gland that is firm, but is nontender.

498. The answer is a. (*South-Paul, pp 443–461.*) Primary hypothyroidism is common, usually a result of Hashimoto's thyroiditis or after Graves' disease. In this case, the TSH would be elevated, and the free T3 and T4 would be low. Secondary hypothyroidism is related to hypothalamic or pituitary dysfunction. Iodine deficiency is a cause of primary hypothyroidism. Subclinical hypothyroidism is when the TSH is elevated, but the T3 and T4 are normal. Thyroid resistance would present with the TSH, T3, and T4 all being elevated.

499. The answer is c. (*South-Paul, pp 443–461.*) Thyroid receptor antibodies are very specific, and differentiate Graves' disease from other causes of hyperthyroidism. The TSH and free thyroid hormones are nonspecific, and only identify hyperthyroidism. Radionucleotide imaging is helpful in Graves', showing diffuse uptake, but is not necessarily specific. Thyroid ultrasonography can identify nodules, but is also a nonspecific test for differentiating causes of hyperthyroidism.

500. The answer is b. (*South-Paul, pp 443–461.*) Once a thyroid nodule is found, the next step in the workup is radionucleotide imaging. If a nodule takes up radiotracer, it is termed a "hot" nodule. Colloidal cysts and tumors do not take up tracer and are "cold" nodules. Therefore, "hot" nodules are more likely benign. Neurofibromas would also be "cold." Definitive diagnosis can be made through needle aspiration.

Bibliography

Barton J, Branch WT. Approach to the Patient with Vertigo. http://www.utdol.com/utd/content/topic.do?topicKey=genneuro/2118&type=A&selectedTitle=2~29. Accessed 8/21/2006.

Brennan T, Blank L, Cohen J, et al. Medical Professionalism in the New Millennium: A Physician Charter. *Ann Intern Med.* 2002;136:243–246.

Castells MC. Insect Stings. http://www.utdol.com/utd/content/topic.do?topicKey=allergy/2070&type=A&selectedTitle=2~12. Accessed 8/26/2006.

Drucker DJ, Nauck MA. The incretin system: glucagon-like peptide-1 receptor agonists and dipeptidyl peptidase-4 inhibitors in type 2 diabetes. *Lancet.* Nov 11, 2006;368(9548):1696–1705.

Fletcher SW, Barton MB. Evaluation of Breast Lumps and Abnormal Mammograms. http://www.utdol.com/utd/content/topic.do?topicKey=genr_med/43947&type=A&selectedTitle=1~8. Accessed 8/27/06.

Goldberg E, Chopra S. Diagnostic Approach to the Patient with Cirrhosis. http://www.utdol.com/utd/content/topic.do?topicKey=cirrhosi/6052&view=print. Accessed 11/28/2006.

Goldstein AO, Goldstein BG. Dermatophyte (Tinea) Infections. http://www.utdol.com/utd/content/topic.do?topicKey=pri_derm/5934&type=A&selectedTitle=1~5. Accessed 8/27/2006.

Hinnen D, Nielsen LL, Waninger A, et al. Incretin Mimetics and DPP-IV Inhibitors: New Paradigms for the Treatment of Type 2 Diabetes. *J Am Board Fam Med.* 2006;19:612–620.

Koski RR. Practical Review of Oral Antihyperglycemic Agents for Type 2 Diabetes Mellitus. *Diabetes Educ.* 2006;32:869–876.

Light RW. Primary Spontaneous Pneumothorax in Adults. http://www.utdol.com/utd/content/topic.do?topicKey=pleurdis/9228. Accessed 12/6/2006.

MacFarlane DP, Fisher M. Thiazolidinediones in Patients with Diabetes Mellitus and Heart Failure: Implications of Emerging Data. *Am J Cardiovasc Drugs.* 2006;6(5):297–304.

Mahutte NG, Duleba AJ. Evaluating Diagnostic Tests. http://www.utdol.com/utd/content/topic.do?topicKey=genr_med/28312&type=A&selectedTitle=1~5. Accessed 12/6/2006.

Meisel JL. Diagnostic Approach to Chest Pain in Adults. http://www.utdol.com/utd/content/topic.do?topicKey=pri_card/2346&type=A&selectedTitle=1~87. Accessed 12/6/2006.

Mengel MB, Schweibert LP (eds). *Family Medicine Ambulatory Care and Prevention, 4th edition.* New York, Lange Medical Books/McGraw-Hill; 2005.

Penner RM, Majumdar SR. Diagnostic Approach to Abdominal Pain in Adults. http://www.utdol.com/utd/content/topic.do?topicKey=pri_gast/4946&type=A&selectedTitle=1~181. Accessed 8/7/2006.

Rakel RE, Bope ET (eds). *Conn's Current Therapy 2006.* Philadelphia, PA, Saunders/Elsevier; 2006.

Recommendations for clinical preventative services. The American Academy of Family Physicians. http://www.aafp.org/online/en/home/clinical/exam/k-o.html. Accessed 10/03/2006.

Rosner B. *Fundamentals of Biostatistics, 5th edition.* Pacific Grove, CA, Duxbury; 2000.

Shadlen MF, Larson EB. Evaluation of Cognitive Impairment and Dementia. http://www.utdol.com/utd/content/topic.do?topicKey=nuroegen/6698&type=A&selectedTitle=5~42. Accessed 2/25/2007.

Shammash JB, Kimmel SE, Morgan JP. Estimation of Cardiac Risk Prior to Noncardiac Surgery. http://www.utdol.com/utd/content/topic.do?topicKey=periart/7170&type=A&selectedTitle=6~58. Accessed 12/3/2006.

Smetana GW. Preoperative Medical Evaluation of the Healthy Patient. http://www.utdol.com/utd/content/topic.do?topicKey=med_cons/6474&view=print. Accessed 11/30/2006.

South-Paul JE, Matheny SC, Lewis EL (eds). *Current Diagnosis and Treatment in Family Medicine.* New York, Lange Medical Books/McGraw-Hill, 2004.

Swaroop Vege S, Chari ST. Clinical Manifestations and Diagnosis of Acute Pancreatitis. http://www.utdol.com/utd/content/topic.do?topicKey=pancdis/7667&type=A&selectedTitle=1~134. Accessed 12/7/2006.

Taylor RB (ed). *Family Medicine Principles and Practice, 6th edition.* New York, Springer; 2003.

Weller PF. Immunizations for Travel. http://www.utdol.com/utd/content/topic.do?topidKey+immunize/6150&view=print. Accessed 11/30/2006.

Wolff K, Johnson RA, Suurmond D (eds). *Fitzpatrick's Color Atlas and Synopsis of Clinical Dermatology, 5th edition.* New York, McGraw-Hill; 2005.

Index